Sexual/Liberation

Síreacht: Longings for Another Ireland is a series of short, topical and provocative texts on controversial issues in contemporary Ireland.

Contributors to the *Síreacht* series come from diverse backgrounds and perspectives but share a commitment to the exposition of what may often be disparaged as utopian ideas, minority perspectives on society, polity and environment, or critiques of received wisdom. Associated with the phrase *ceól síreachtach síde* found in Irish medieval poetry, *síreacht* refers to yearnings such as those evoked by the music of the *aos sí*, the supernatural people of Irish mythology. As the title for this series, we use it to signify longings for and imaginings of a better world in the spirit of the World Social Forums that 'another world is possible'. At the heart of the mythology of the *sí* is the belief that lying beneath this world is the other world. So too these texts address the urgent challenge to imagine potential new societies and relationships, but also to recognise the seeds of these other worlds in what already exists.

Other published titles in the series are

Freedom? by Two Fuse
Commemoration by Heather Laird
Public Sphere by Harry Browne
Money by Conor McCabe
Self by Eilís Ward

The editors of the series, Órla O'Donovan, Fiona Dukelow, Rosie Meade, School of Applied Social Studies and Heather Laird, School of English, University College Cork, welcome suggestions or proposals for consideration as future titles in the series. Please see http://sireacht.ie/ for more information.

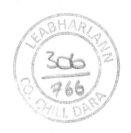

Sexual/Liberation

MICHAEL G. CRONIN

Series Editors:
Órla O'Donovan, Fiona Dukelow,
Rosie Meade and Heather Laird

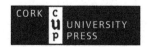

CORK
CUP
UNIVERSITY
PRESS

First published in 2022 by
Cork University Press
Boole Library
University College Cork
Cork T12 ND89
Ireland

Library of Congress number: 2022936355

British Library Cataloguing in Publication Data
A CIP catalogue record for this book is available from the British
Library.

ISBN 9781782055235

Typeset by Studio 10 Design
Printed by Hussar Books in Poland

Cover image © Shutterstock.com

CONTENTS

Figures   vii

Acknowledgements   ix

Introduction   1

Equality   13

Vulnerability   47

Revolution   69

Liberation   93

Hope   111

Notes and References   131

Bibliography   143

Index   149

Figures

Figure 1   Joe Caslin, 'The Claddagh Embrace'   112

Figure 2   Joe Caslin, 'Ar Scáth a Chéile a
            Mhaireann na Daoine'   113

Figure 3   Joe Caslin, 'The Volunteers –
            Collins Barracks'   115

Acknowledgements

Warm thanks to Órla O'Donovan, Fiona Dukelow, Heather Laird and Rosie Meade, editors of the 'Síreacht: Longings for another Ireland' series, for their enthusiasm, encouragement and patient guidance. Reading Heather's brilliant contribution to the series, *Commemoration*, was the initial spark for writing this book.

Once upon a time I worked for the magazine *GCN*, where I first engaged with the problem of how to think and write politically about sexuality. They may disagree with some, or indeed all, of what I write here, but I gratefully salute inspiring comrades from those days: Deborah Ballard, Brian Finnegan, Ciaran Nolan, Stephen Meyler, Ailbhe Smyth, Tonie Walsh.

I have continued to wrestle with that problem while teaching in the Department of English at Maynooth University and am greatly indebted to students and colleagues in the department and the university. Joe Cleary, Sinéad Kennedy and Emer Nolan have been invaluable friends. Thanks for their ongoing support and love to Deirdre, Sandra and, as always, Tony.

The outstanding work of David Alderson and the late Alan Sinfield enriches and incites my thinking about these questions beyond measure. Cathal Kerrigan's contribution to radical and liberationist politics in Ireland is a powerful exemplar.

My thanks to Joe Caslin for permission to reproduce the images of his murals, including Peter Grogan's photograph.

A version of section three was previously published as 'Pain, Pleasure and Revolution: The body in Roger Casement's writings' in *The Body in Pain in Irish Literature and Culture* (Palgrave, 2016); my thanks to the editors: Fionnuala Dillane, Naomi McAreavey and Emilie Pine. Parts of section five, and some shorter segments, are extracted from my *Revolutionary Bodies: Homoeroticism and the political imagination in Irish writing* (Manchester University Press, 2022).

Introduction

In January 2015, the then minister for health, Leo Varadkar, was interviewed by Miriam O'Callaghan on her RTÉ radio show *Miriam Meets*. During their conversation, Varadkar spoke publicly for the first time about being gay. As is well known, in June 2017 he was elected as leader of the Fine Gael party, and subsequently elected as taoiseach in the Dáil.

The election to that office of the biracial, openly gay son of an immigrant – his father is from India – indexed the scale of demographic, social and cultural change in the Irish republic since Leo Varadkar was born in 1979. At the same time, this event foregrounded in interesting ways the political question of how we might conceptualise such historical transformations. Analysing the media coverage of Varadkar's career, Páraic Kerrigan and Maria Pramaggiore note that journalists from other countries celebrated his election, as leader of what the *New York Post* somewhat anachronistically labelled a 'devoutly Catholic country', as an unalloyed symbol of Irish modernisation. *Time* magazine's subsequent profile of the new taoiseach – the cover story for that issue –

asserted that his election cemented the republic's place as 'an island at the centre of the world'.[1] Progressive social change is thus equated with neoliberal globalisation; 'openness' towards sexual and other forms of diversity in the culture symbolically aligned with 'openness' to financialised global capital in the economy. Kerrigan and Pramaggiore contrast the celebratory tone of this coverage with homophobic undertones in the Irish media's response to later episodes in Varadkar's career as taoiseach. Most notably, reporting and commentary during an absurd, confected 'controversy' about his attendance at a Kylie Minogue concert in 2018 traded in homophobic and misogynistic stereotypes about gay men, pop music and fandom to undermine Varadkar's authority.

In their analysis, Kerrigan and Pramaggiore are as sceptical about Varadkar's international reception as a political 'homohero' as they are critical of the homophobia in the local press.[2] Like some forms of liberal feminism, the 'homohero' narrative situates its antihomophobic commitments within an unquestioning adherence to individualism. In this view, exemplary individual achievement, rather than collective mobilisation, is the only imagined route to progressive change. This is a conception of pluralism in which the prevailing social order is diversified but thereby consolidated rather than transformed; David Alderson terms this the 'diversified dominant' characteristic of neoliberalism.[3]

This binary of homoheroic and homophobic media responses to Varadkar was complicated by a third perspective identified by Kerrigan and Pramaggiore. This was scepticism about his progressive credentials from within the Irish LGBT (Lesbian, Gay, Bisexual and Transgender) political movement; a position neatly encapsulated in one arresting headline from *GCN*: 'Leo Varadkar Will Be as Helpful to the Gays as Margaret Thatcher Was to Women'.[4] In the years since 2015 Varadkar has softened some of his conservative views, most notably on abortion, women's reproductive rights and repealing the eighth amendment. Nevertheless, as the Thatcher analogy implies, his politics exemplify the affinities and connections between neoconservatism and neoliberalism that came to characterise the dominant political rationality in Western democracies during Varadkar's lifetime.

As the political philosopher Wendy Brown argues, neoconservatism and neoliberalism are not identical or interchangeable; one is a market-political rationality with a business model of the state, and the other a moral-political rationality with a theological model of the state.[5] Nevertheless, there are convergences between them, as, for instance, when neoliberal policies for weakening labour rights and welfare supports are framed in moral terms; thus Varadkar's notorious promise to lead a political party for early risers, implying that laziness rather than *laissez-faire* is the primary cause of un-employment (and precarious employment).[6] Moreover,

Brown argues, during the last four decades the articulation between these divergent forms of political rationality has undermined liberal democracy. As she notes, those on the left need not uncritically endorse liberal democracy to be concerned at its morphing into something more authoritarian and less democratic. Brown identifies the key elements in this process of what she terms de-democratisation. These include: the devaluation of political autonomy, as democracy is equated with formal rights, especially property rights, rather than active citizenship; the transformation of political problems into individual problems with market solutions; the production of the consumer-citizen as available to a heavy degree of governance and authority.[7] As we will see, the political objective of securing access to legal marriage for same-sex couples, termed 'marriage equality' in Ireland, conforms with this pattern to a surprisingly high degree.

Evidently, the *GCN* writers were more alert to the actual content of Varadkar's politics than were promoters of the homoheroic narrative. They reiterate that his politics rather than his identity is more consequential when evaluating his potential to be such a homohero. The writers' critique is more sustained and nuanced than the editor's headline, especially since the headline actually registers the same conception of the relationship between sexuality and politics as the homoheroic narrative from which the writers are dissenting. The charge that Varadkar will not be 'helpful to the gays' implies a disappointed expectation that, as an openly gay politician, he ought to be. This view illustrates a minoritarian form of politics, which I will be critiquing in this essay. Just as importantly, this expectation is underpinned by a confident assumption that 'the gays' are a homogeneous group bound by a common set of interests. This precludes the possibility that his policies could further the interests of some affluent 'gays' while disimproving the lives of other 'gays'.[8] Again, this illustrates the problem with a political conception of sexuality as autonomous from class relations, which will also be the subject of critique below.

This discursive figure called 'Leo Varadkar' – which for convenience we might provisionally categorise as distinct from the private man and political figure bearing that name – usefully illustrates the concerns animating this book. These divergent responses to an openly gay politician illustrate that in the dreamworld of late capitalism the 'gay man' is an ideologically mobile figure to which politically, and affectively, contradictory perspectives adhere. As the homophobic tropes rehearsed by some Irish journalists when writing about 'Leo Varadkar' attest, the discursive gay man presents a threatening figure, potentially undermining normative structures of gender, family and patriarchy. He might, for instance, blur clear lines of gender identity through his 'unmanly' investment in the stylised femininity embodied in the persona of a singing star like Kylie. Yet, it is precisely this same threat which the discursive gay man presents to the dominant gender and sexual order that is for others a source of energising hope. For the *GCN* writers, for instance, this hopeful belief in the emancipatory possibilities of sexual identity underpins their clear disenchantment with the present reformist reality of mainstream LGBT politics embodied in the homoheroic 'Leo Varadkar'. For the *Time* writer, this figure also embodies hope, but of a different kind. This is not a yearning for revolutionary transformation but, on the contrary, a longing for stability – the inclusion of such homoheros into the dominant capitalist order, it is hoped, being one way in which everything might change to stay the same.

Leo Varadkar's election was neither revolutionary nor regressive. It was neither the apotheosis of transformative social change, the homoheroic account, nor a great betrayal of the transformative potential promised by politicised sexual identities, the 'failing the gays' account. His election was symbolically significant for Irish society and emotionally resonant for many lesbian and gay people. Above all, his election indexed the remarkable achievements of Irish social movements since the 1970s – most notably feminism and the lesbian and gay movement – and the hard-won evolution of more tolerant social norms and a more hospitable, diverse society. That he could, as an openly gay man, become taoiseach was a victory for those movements since they had striven to create the conditions where this was possible. But that he became taoiseach was also a defeat for those same movements. It signalled just how marginalised and suppressed the radical liberationist currents within those movements have become. As *Time* magazine approvingly registered, Varadkar's election exemplified the hegemony of neoliberal political rationality. Far from representing the achievement of liberation, his election represented the ascendancy of a debased idea of freedom as consumer choice, and a social order in which human freedom must always be subordinated to the freedom of global capital to extract profit at any human or ecological cost. The world-view embodied by 'Leo Varadkar' is the dominant world-view in contemporary capitalism, and rather than a heroic ideal to which we should aspire, it is, on the contrary, imperative to oppose and defeat that world-view – nothing less than the survival of democracy and of human life depends on the outcome of that struggle.

As I outline below, *Sexual/Liberation* addresses those paradoxes of sexual freedom in late capitalism encapsulated in this story of Ireland's first gay taoiseach. I address that topic from the standpoint of trying to imagine a revolutionary form of sexual liberation beyond the present objective of achieving sexual equality within a grossly unequal social order. This is an essay in five sections, each one exploring either a political objective (equality; revolution; liberation) or a politically mobilising affect (vulnerability; hope). As with 'Leo Varadkar', my discussion of these themes is propelled by reflections on images and discursive figures circulating in contemporary Irish culture. These images are of gay men, the male body and homoerotic passion, and in the first section I explain my political as well as personal reasons for this specific focus. As I hope to make clear, this is not an essay about gay men and their distinctive experiences but about how our culture thinks and feels about the 'gay man' as a discursive figure. My motivating question is not 'how can gay men be free from homophobia?' but 'how can our society be radically transformed, and liberation achieved for everybody?'

The first section critiques the demand for equality, around which the campaign for same-sex marriage rights mobilised so successfully in 2015. I develop this critique by contrasting two visual representations of male intimacy: advertising for wedding services, and digital self-portraits posted online by men engaging in sex work. Together these images foreground for us the limitations and paradoxes of equality as a political objective. Or, more precisely, 'equality' – the parasitic neoliberal deformation of that otherwise politically desirable outcome of equality; that form of 'equality' so familiarly institutionalised as a commitment to EDI (equality, diversity and inclusion) by corporations and organisations, including universities, whose actual treatment of workers perpetuates stark inequalities.

Moving on, I adapt the concept of vulnerability from Judith Butler's work, taking up her challenge to encounter human vulnerability as an affective wellspring for radical political mobilisation. As a politically mobilising affect, vulnerability can be favourably compared with injury, which is, I argue – taking my coordinates from Wendy Brown – the primary affect animating contemporary identity politics. By contrast with the radical universalism of vulnerability, injury is individualist, enclosed and self-defeating. Thinking about how Declan Flynn, who was killed in a homophobic attack in Dublin in 1982, is currently memorialised as an exemplary victim of homophobia, and how the repercussions of his death are now interpreted as initiating the journey towards marriage equality, offers a suggestive route towards grasping that politically operative distinction between vulnerability and injury.

Remembering a different historical figure, Roger Casement, frames the 'revolution' section. Casement wrote about the vulnerability of the human body to the violence of extractive capitalism, making powerful use of that style of writing to develop a revolutionary, anti-imperialist challenge to an exploitative global order. He also wrote about the male body as a site of pleasure and delight, and that too, I argue, can inspire the anti-capitalist and revolutionary imagination. That section ends by contrasting different modes of commemorating Casement a century after his execution by the British imperial state. One mode focuses on Casement's hybrid identities, transforming him into a symbol of the diversified dominant in late capitalist Ireland and a reassuring icon of the present. By contrast, I advocate a mode of remembrance which focuses on Casement's radicalising encounter with the bodies of the dispossessed;

a mode of remembrance which strives to find in his insurrectionary vision a pathway to a transformed future.

These distinctions – vulnerability/injury; body/identity – merge with another pairing in the following section: liberation/reformism. A photograph of a group of gay men defiantly, and joyously, marching on Dublin's O'Connell Street in 1984, from the archives of the Dublin Lesbian and Gay Collective, encourages us to imaginatively recapture a paradoxical moment in the history of the Irish lesbian and gay movement; a time defined by tragedy, loss, grief and demoralisation that was simultaneously a time defined by radical energies and vibrant mobilisation around revolutionary goals. Noting the subsequent occlusion of those revolutionary and liberationist currents in the prevailing homoheroic narrative of Irish queer history prompts us to reflect on the affinities between the ascendency of lesbian and gay reformism and of neoliberal political rationality. More positively, though, it might also encourage us to explore that occluded liberationist current more energetically and encounter again its intellectual origins in Herbert Marcuse's writing.

This essay ends where all revolutionary politics begins – with hope. As Ernst Bloch argued, hope is indispensable for any revolutionary politics. Just like institutionalised 'equality', a tamed, commodified version of hope has been assimilated into neoliberal political rationality, with its promise of unfettered affluence and self-actualisation for the entrepreneurially adept subject.

By contrast, as I outline in the final section, Bloch argued that cultivating revolutionary hope demands a different style of temporal reasoning than the linear progressive time demanded by capitalism. This requires encountering the future as an open possibility, while being responsive to the revolutionary dreams of a transformed future we inherit from the past.[9] Likewise, Bloch identified the necessity of what he termed 'guiding images' of a liberated humanity, which help us to hopefully imagine what freedom might look like. For these reasons, Bloch argues, art is essential to the cultivation of political hope. In the final section I take Joe Caslin's murals, and especially his style of depicting male bodies and male intimacy, as a good example of politically hopeful art in contemporary Irish culture. In almost every respect, Caslin's art resists the dominant neoliberal rationality: collective and collaborative rather than individualist; eluding monetisation and commodification by the 'art market'; reclaiming public space for the commons. This essay ends with Caslin's art because it belongs among those creative practices which are 'located at the threshold of politics and aesthetics; practices that generate spaces where alternative social forms can emerge, and where unscripted futures can be imagined'.[10]

Equality

exual/Liberation addresses a universal topic from a particular standpoint. That universal is the quality or condition of sexual freedom in late capitalist society. In late-twentieth-century Ireland sexual freedom was primarily defined as freedom from restrictive regulation by the state and from the oppressive hegemonic norms of Catholic sexual 'morality'. There are compelling historical and political reasons for the salience of this conception of sexual freedom in Irish politics.

The feminist and gay and lesbian social movements that emerged in Ireland in the 1970s constituted a broad struggle, fought on various fronts, to assert the autonomy of individuals over their body and enhance their freedom. Necessarily women were to the forefront, since the key issues had most immediate effect on their health, well-being and liberty, issues such as: access to birth control and termination; introducing welfare support for single mothers and challenging their stigmatisation; reforming the archaic marriage laws; legalising divorce.

In the 1970s this emergent movement confronted a then still dominant ideology, which combined capitalism with a fusion of Catholicism and conservative nationalism. Since the post-Famine decades of the mid-nineteenth century this ideological formation had placed an oppressive emphasis on controlling the body, the emotions and all expressions of human sexual needs and pleasures.[11] Maintaining such control was held to be a moral but also an economic and political imperative. With the creation of the two confessional states after partition in 1922 the cultural stress on such control was given further legislative force. In its first two decades the Free State kept the legislation banning abortion and sex between men (criminalised as 'gross indecency' since 1885) inherited from the imperial parliament in Westminster, while adding a comprehensive ban on birth control, and information on it, and a constitutional ban on divorce.

Thus, a central objective of Irish feminism, and liberal and progressive politics more broadly, since the 1970s has been to dismantle the architecture of containment, to use Jim Smith's phrase, consolidated in the decades after independence. That architecture encompassed the physical infrastructure of Magdalene asylums, mother and baby homes and industrial schools, where those in breach of the sexual ethic of the post-independence society could be confined, punished and kept out of view. As Smith argues, this physical architecture of containment was inseparable from the ideological and discursive architecture through which those institutions were administered, sustained and, crucially, normalised.[12] As I write, the debate about the *Final Report of the Commission of Investigation into Mother and Baby Homes* indicates how Irish society is still grappling, with only partial success, to confront the human suffering endured by working-class women and children incarcerated in those institutions, and how the women who suffered in those places are still fighting to have their voices count.[13]

Now, in the twenty-first century, two pillars of that ideological formation, which was hegemonic in Ireland from independence to the 1970s, have been eroded and undermined. The authority of the Catholic Church as the arbiter of sexual morality and ethics, and promoter of the social regulation of sexual conduct, has been fundamentally challenged by progressive social movements while simultaneously being undermined by its own institutional actions in covering up the sexual abuse of children. Likewise, conservative nationalism has, to a large degree, lost its hold over how we now imagine the imagined community of the Irish nation. But capitalism, the third pillar of that formation, is as hegemonic now as it has ever been in Irish history. We need look no further than the ongoing housing crisis to recognise how the rights of property still triumph over all human and social needs, just as they did in the decades after independence. It is for this reason that, while still striving to understand and remember the painful legacy of how sexuality, and specifically women's sexuality, was oppressively controlled in Catholic-nationalist Ireland, we also need a new framework for understanding how human sexuality is being regulated differently in contemporary neoliberal Ireland.

One starting point for developing such a framework is to challenge the conventional idea of sexual freedom as an autonomous type of political objective. My title indexes this by focusing on liberation rather than freedom, with the punctuation inviting us to speculate on how we might connect the ideal of revolutionary liberation with those dimensions of human experience denoted by the word 'sexual'. Critical reflection on, and political mobilisation around, sexual freedom is inseparable from critical reflection on, and political mobilisation around, freedom as such.

From the twentieth century our culture has inherited a powerfully compelling model of sexuality as a natural instinct – as impulses, desires, libidinal energies – that is at the definitional core of who we are and woven into the fabric of our identity. In this view, desire is heavily constrained and controlled by the repressive force of society. By contrast, as Rosemary Hennessy argues, a materialist conception of human sexuality asks us to consider sexuality not in terms of sexual desire, but more broadly as the human potential for sensation and affect – what Ann Ferguson terms 'sex-affective energy' – that is a key component of all social relations.[14] In this view, our need for love, intimacy, affection and pleasure – including some of our darker, troubling pleasures – would form one distinctive component on an elastic, historically contingent continuum of needs; needs that are corporeal, essential to physical survival, but not 'natural', since these needs can only ever be met in and through social relations.

Under capitalism, the production of surplus value, profit, is accompanied by what Hennessy calls the 'outlawing' of human needs. The 'price' paid to a worker for his or her labour excludes many of the worker's potentials and needs as the unnamed price of the exchange. One form this outlawing of needs takes is the gender ideology that displaces the meeting of human needs onto the domestic labour of feeding, clothing and caring that is marked, and devalued, as woman's 'natural' role and either unpaid or underpaid. Another form is the commodification of consciousness through which sensation and affect get separated from the meeting of human needs, either directly as the abuse of workers' bodies and minds in the pursuit of profit or indirectly 'through forms of consciousness that abstract mind from body, public from private, ways of knowing from their historical material conditions'.[15] For Hennessy a salient instance of this latter dynamic was the emergence of our contemporary sex-gender system from the late nineteenth century onwards. This consolidation of sexuality into a matrix of identities, she argues, 'reified the human potential for sensation and affect ... in the process of reifying consciousness into forms of identity, whole areas of human affective potential are effectively outlawed'.

Another way of conceptualising this difference between sexual freedom and sexual liberation is Herbert Marcuse's distinction between 'sexuality' and 'Eros', which I explain further in section four. In *One-Dimensional Man* (1964) Marcuse identified the socially sanctioned release of repressed sexuality as an emerging phenomenon in modern capitalist societies. For Marcuse, this liberalisation of sexual norms and relaxing of taboos was entirely different from sexual liberation as he conceptualised it. Liberation did not require the lifting of societal and psychic repression but the transformation of sexuality, as currently understood and lived, into the condition of freedom beyond alienation that Marcuse termed Eros. For Marcuse, 'sexuality' describes a human instinct concentrated on genital activity and reproduction, and which is, in Marcuse's terms, sacramentalised – granted social sanction and symbolic meaning, 'humanised', through mediating rituals such as marriage. Those sacramentalising rituals are impelled by the idea that human sexuality is inherently impure. While this idea was historically rooted in a Judeo-Christian *Weltanschauung*, Marcuse reiterates that the secularising effects of capitalism changed the terms in which we frame the impurity of sexuality – 'sinful' displaced by 'unhealthy' – but that sacramentalism still underpins the type of sexual freedom granted to us in late capitalism. 'Eros' does not describe liberated sexuality, but the creation of an entirely new way of inhabiting our bodies in which the desires, needs and pleasures currently concentrated on 'sexuality' are dispersed across the body and inhere in all social relations. What 'Eros' means is difficult to articulate, but that is because it names a form of liberation which we cannot yet 'know' and can only imagine – hence, for Marcuse, the vital function of art in helping us to develop a revolutionary imagination. Crucially, unlike the achievement of sexual freedom within the existing structures of capitalist society, the transformation of sexuality into Eros will only be possible through the revolutionary transformation of all social relations, not just those we currently think of as 'sexual' or 'personal'. The transformation of sexuality into Eros will be one essential element of the revolutionary transformation of capitalism into democratic socialism. As Marcuse recognised, and this is a vital insight of twentieth-century radical feminist, Marxist and anti-colonial thought, a revolution confined to institutions, to economic and political structures, is doomed to failure to the degree that it neglects to revolutionise human consciousness.

In late capitalism, the sanctioned release of repressed sexuality has integrated the creative potential of human erotic energies more securely into the dominant system, thus restricting while expanding human freedom. For instance, the immense profitability of the globalised porn industry alongside the pervasive incorporation of porn tropes into 'legitimate' advertising is just one obvious illustration of this development. As Marcuse foresaw, these were developments in capitalist society which 'extend liberty while intensifying domination'.[16] From the perspective of women in contemporary society, that the form of sexual freedom offered by late capitalism might be a form of coercive unfreedom is less a remarkable critical insight than a grimly familiar description of reality. For instance, the testimony recorded during the trial of four men accused of raping and sexually assaulting a young woman in Belfast during spring 2018 graphically illustrated the endemic misogyny, and celebration of sexualised violence against women, which characterises the pornified culture in which men and women are interpellated as sexual subjects, and which women must precariously navigate.[17]

In what follows I am addressing this universal topic, sexual freedom in late capitalism, from a very specific perspective; that is, a critical meditation on the circulation of images of gay men in contemporary Irish culture. There are a number of reasons for this emphasis on images – or discursive figures – and on gay men. One reason is personal; I am struck by the historical synchronicity that I was born in 1974, the year that the Irish Gay Rights Movement was founded. And so, tuning into, and critically reflecting on, Irish culture's images of gay men has been central to my emotional, sexual, intellectual and political formation. This has been propelled by understanding what my society imagines 'gay men' to be, but also by incorporating and resisting how that society defines me as subject and citizen. I recall a particularly odd distillation of this psycho-political dynamic from 23 May 2015. Watching the jubilant crowds gathered at Dublin Castle celebrating the success of the referendum to enshrine the right to marriage for same-sex couples in the Irish constitution, I experienced a discombobulating access of affective dissonance. I was deeply moved to be accepted by a society whose acceptance I had never consciously sought or desired, a society whose dominant neoliberal values I find, in almost every respect, inhumane and abhorrent.

Another reason for this specific approach might be categorised as 'professional'; though, as anyone working in the neoliberal university knows, it is imperative to resist the managerial regulation and intellectual enfeeblement enacted by that concept – and its cognates: 'specialism'/'expertise' – if intellectual work of any real value is to be achieved. Nevertheless, I teach and write as a literary critic; in other words, one who evaluates the political and cultural significance of the fictional stories which a society tells itself. Moreover, in doing that work I find the 'reflection model', as Raymond Williams termed it, inadequate for grasping the active and dynamic ideological 'work' which literature and visual culture enact.[18] Fictional stories and cultural images are politically important not for their depiction of the society as it is – the artwork as mirror in which society sees its reflection – but for the insight they offer into the political unconscious of that society. Cultural images of 'gay men' tell us very little about actually-existing men who identify as gay in all the variegated complexity of their lives and material conditions. But such images offer us a great deal of insight into the political imaginary – the values, norms, anxieties and ideological contradictions – of the society in which those images circulate.

The third reason for adopting this particular standpoint might be termed 'political'; assuming that the 'political' can be so neatly distinguished from other spheres of our creative and affective lives, a distinction in itself ideological and de-politicising. Simply put, a critical understanding of how images of gay men circulate in the contemporary political imaginary can potentially sharpen our capacity to imagine sexual liberation for all. To reiterate, the object of inquiry here is not the historical and social *experiences* of gay men but the circulation of images, ways of imagining gay men, in late capitalism. And images of gay men circulate very distinctively within what Walter Benjamin termed the phantasmagorias of capitalism – that hallucinatory, incessant flow of images and sensations that characterises consumer society.[19]

In the twenty-first century the discursive image of the gay man, or 'homosexual', as a threatening and subversive figure, inherited by us from the nineteenth and twentieth centuries, is still part of the conservative political imaginary. This is true within Western democracies but is more viscerally so in countries such as Hungary, Poland, Russia and certain Middle-Eastern and African states, for instance, where this figure is being actively mobilised to incite legal persecution and violence against queer people.[20] But from within the perspective of the neoliberal world-view now hegemonic in Western democracies, such as Ireland, this figure of the gay man as 'other' seems residual in two senses.

Firstly, in this dominant world-view homophobia is positioned as a residual phenomenon. That is, as an effect of pre-modern modes of thought and subjectivity – religion, nationalism, despotism, irrationalism – persistently infecting an otherwise rational, secular, democratic and cosmopolitan body politic. In this view, homophobia is considered an epiphenomenon which it is unnecessary to conceptualise as a political problem within, or specific to, capitalism. Thus, it is considered unnecessary, for instance, to register that some of the most virulent political mobilisation of homophobia is currently located in states where extractive capitalism is most exploitative and kleptocratic.

Secondly, the idea of the gay man as threatening seems residual in a culture where the most familiar imagery of gay men situates these figures at the definitional core, rather than the stigmatised periphery, of normative subjectivity – of what it is to be recognisably human. In its most overtly 'political' variant, this image of the gay man is a heroic figure representing an embattled minority which successfully staked its claim to recognition. Not just heroic but redemptive, since the extension of such recognition affirms and endorses the prevailing values and norms of that society. This is not just political but politically affective; we can all 'feel good' about what has been achieved. In a more depoliti-cising variant, this imaginary gay man embodies an ideal version of the entrepreneurial neoliberal subject; that imaginary 'free' subject would be wholly responsible for their own self-care, rationally making choices to maximise the benefits accruing to them and striving to embody a conception of 'success' narrowly defined by affluence and by the illusion of competitive autonomy. This is the 'gay man' as embodiment of what the collaborative writers known as Two Fuse term the 'scripted practices of freedom' promoted by our 'Enterprise Society'.[21]

Let us begin then with a photograph of two men dancing. These handsome men are in their late twenties or early thirties and dressed in tuxedos. Their dancing is formal – their pose suggests a waltz – but warmly af-fectionate: clasped hands; cheeks gently touching. The room in which they dance has flower petals scattered on the floorboards and lit candles on a table in the back-ground. A small group of well-dressed people watch the dancing couple, and a photographer stands to the side with his camera lens directed towards them. The cap-tured moment is at once intimate and public. Given these visual clues, the slogans alongside the image are not entirely surprising: 'Your Wedding Dance' and 'Make it Magical!', along with an invitation to 'Book a class now at Viva School of Dance'.

This half-page advert was published in the October 2019 issue of *GCN*, which the editorial described as the 'ninth annual wedding issue'.[22] The issue includes a series of interviews with same-sex couples about their lives together – but heavily concentrated on how they had planned and celebrated their weddings or were planning to do so. These interviews were surrounded by advertising and advertorial from hotels and wedding venues, along with florists, wine suppliers and charities (promoting charitable contributions as 'wedding favours'). In addition, there was advertorial copy written by an estate agent (whose company also placed a paid advert) offering advice to 'first-time buyers'.

This *GCN* 'wedding issue' literalises Marcuse's observation that, in the form of capitalist society taking shape as he wrote, 'sexual liberty is harmonised with profitable conformity'.[23] It is tempting to use a colonial metaphor here. The capitalist market is moving into a new territory and striving to extract profit from the previously untapped resource of same-sex desires and relationships. However, as Katherine Sender notes in her analysis of marketing aimed at lesbians and gay men in the United States, that view presumes a fixed or static conception of identity and disregards the dynamic, creative and relational activity of identity-making. As Stuart Hall argued, identities are 'points of temporary attachment to the subject positions which discursive practices construct for us all'.[24] Thus, as Sender observes, 'sexual identity is produced in the spaces between subjects and discourses, readers and texts, consumers and things'.[25] For that reason, it is necessary to approach marketing not as neutral activity by 'rational' actors but as among the various discourses which are actively constituting and shaping sexual and other identities. Marketing, as Sender observes, 'does not merely represent gay and lesbian people, but produces recognisable – and sellable – definitions of what it means to be gay or lesbian'.[26]

The recurring imagery in the *GCN* special issue conflates the visible performance of marital 'happiness' for lesbian and gay people with the performance of 'success', where such success is in turn conflated with affluence. This is conveyed most blatantly in the framing of the estate agent advertorial; that unacknowledged assumption that the typical readership of a *GCN* 'wedding issue' can afford to buy a home in a society where meeting our human need for shelter is so starkly subordinated to a profit-seeking market logic. However, it is captured much more affectingly and poignantly in the 'Viva School of Dance' advertisement, reiterating the cruel paradox that in this economy of romance spontaneous affection will 'fail' if it is not assiduously and expensively rehearsed.

However, it is crucial to stress that those stories of shared love recounted by the couples in the articles are not in any way invalidated or exposed as inauthentic by the surrounding advertisements and advertorial. On the contrary, it is precisely the profound depth of feeling – reservoirs of human need and relationality – expressed in those stories that the neoliberal market strives to reify, commodify and profitably monetise. To put this another way, we could say that the 'wedding issue' stages a dichotomy between two distinct, contradictory but equally resonant meanings of marriage.

One is marriage as it exists now. Firstly, marriage as a social ritual with deep roots in the sacramentalism of Judeo-Christian and post-Enlightenment bourgeois culture. The historical development of that ritual was powerfully propelled by a long-standing and persistent belief that, as David Alderson summarises, 'sexual pleasure stands in need of redemption, whether conceived in religious or humanistic terms, and that this endows the sacramental relationship with a qualitative moral and emotional superiority over all others'.[27] Secondly, marriage as a form of legal contract – again, with deep roots in pre-modern aristocratic alliance and modern bourgeois property rights – which is expected to counterbalance the inherent instability and disorientating flux engendered by capitalism. In its contemporary form, this contract conceptualises human relationships as aggregative and individualist rather than relational and collective; two individuals merge to function as an individual. As Alison Shonkwiller argues, 'the modern family serves as a larger new unit of "selfhood" within the terms of liberal individualism. In this sense, the development of the gay family cannot be separated from the development of the family in general as a way to organise consumption'.[28] The intensified privatisation of neoliberal culture, and the dismantling of the socialised supports of welfare capitalism in recent decades, makes the family the location to which we are

increasingly forced to turn to sustain ourselves, to negotiate the marketplace and to manage our lives with some
degree of security. Thirdly, marriage and the family as a
privatised resource for the reproduction of labour and
the principal mechanism through which the physical and
affective work of sustaining human life is naturalised as
the responsibility of women in bourgeois gender ideology. Marriage as a social institution which facilitates
and naturalises that situation in which, as Alison Phipps
summarises, 'women's work is not viewed as real work: it
exists in the realm of "love", not money'.[29]

This is marriage as it is now. But the hopes and desires
so many of us invest in the idea of marriage clearly
transcend this reality. Marriage offers a glimpse of future
possibilities – of what human consciousness might be
like in transformed conditions, where the relations of
production were directed towards the collective meeting
of human needs. The marital ideal and its mediating social
rituals is so emotionally resonant and compelling – and,
conversely, the reality of 'being married' so exhausting
to sustain – because such a variety of 'outlawed' human
needs – from pleasure to shelter – are condensed
within it. The stories from the couples in the *GCN*
'wedding issue' articulate a hopeful faith in the imagined
potentialities emblematised in marriage: potential
forms of human relationship in which human need,
vulnerability and interdependence might be a potent
solvent of self-interested, entrepreneurial individualism
and a source of collective solidarity. In marriage we

glimpse a not-yet-become freedom that is not predicated on the autonomy of the sovereign individual but on the vulnerability of a dependent human body; we glimpse a world where all human relationships resemble what we ideally, and under current conditions unsustainably, expect of marriage.

The tension between marriage as reconciliation to the reality principle of late capitalism and marriage as emblem of utopian possibility was powerfully operative in the campaign for same-sex marriage rights leading to the 2015 referendum. That tension was condensed most obviously around the use of the term 'equality'. Like Leo Varadkar's election, the referendum result presented a complex challenge for any radical sexual politics. The difficulty is to grasp how this political objective was simultaneously progressive and conservative – promoting inclusivity and pluralism while adhering to the prevailing neoliberal political rationality. An inclusive, pluralist and just vision of society prevailed over a vision that was rigid, narrow and intolerant. The majority chose to live in a society that affirms and celebrates love; perhaps realising that such a society will ultimately be a better place for all of its citizens, not only its lesbian and gay citizens.

But the vote also solidified the institution of marriage as the lynchpin of a patriarchal, property-owning society.[30] The conception of equality affirmed in the 'marriage equality' campaign was quite narrowly formalist and contractual. The 'yes' rhetoric conjured a reassuringly neoliberal vision of lesbian and gay households 'equally' free to compete, as privatised units of consumption, and striving to successfully manage their resources. And while the symbolic centrality of family imagery in the 'yes' campaign may have been strategically effective, it also symbolically reinforced a modern pluralised version of sacramentalism. As the philosopher Wendy Brown observed of the campaign for same-sex marriage rights in the United States, we have to confront the 'unspeakable suggestion' that 'gays and lesbians promulgating marriage as the ultimate sanctification of love between two people are biting from the same mythohistorical muffin as anti-gay conservatives declaring marriage to be timeless and transcendent in meaning'.[31]

Securing same-sex marriage rights first developed as a political priority in the United States in the mid-1990s and this development was a consequence of the AIDS crisis. As Melinda Cooper demonstrates, confronted by the appalling failure of the American health system to respond effectively and justly to the needs of HIV-positive people, ACT-UP, along with other militant queer groups, revived radical demands for accessible healthcare and expanded social insurance that had first been articulated by sections of the American left in the 1970s. As Cooper argues, some AIDS activists looked to that tradition to 'imagine a universal system of health insurance that was no longer tied to the old restrictions of the family wage – a system that divorced healthcare coverage from employment and marital status'.[32] However, their campaign was defeated by the welfare 'reforms' of the Clinton administration and, more generally, by 'the increasingly influential ethic of personal and family responsibility associated with neoliberalism'.[33] This prompted an about-turn in LGBT politics in the United States; away from challenging the inhumanity and injustices of privatised healthcare and towards seeking inclusion and protection, through same-sex civil partnership and marriage rights, *within* that unjust system. Here again, the contrasting political rationalities of neoliberalism and neoconservatism converged within the emergent political discourse in favour of same-sex marriage rights: 'if AIDS was the price to pay for irresponsible lifestyle choice, same-sex marriage was now presented as the route to personal (and hence familial) responsibility'.[34]

Strikingly, the cover slogan on the *GCN* marriage issue in October 2019 appears to address just these tensions in the concept of marriage equality: 'Love' over the word 'Equality'. Could this be an exhortation to love the political objective of equality? That is, challenging us to love (value; commit ourselves to) the ideal of a social order where human needs are met, exploitation is absent and freedom and human potentiality find expression. Alternatively, is the challenge to think about the connection between love and equality? What is the political relationship between how we might fulfil those human needs encoded in the word 'love' (nurture, connection, intimacy, pleasure, excitement, glamour, affirmation) and various other, related, human needs? Is love even possible in a social order where the whole spectrum of human needs go unmet for so many, and where the means through which to fulfil those needs are so inequitably distributed? Can there be love where there is no freedom from necessity?

However, this invitation to speculation about equality as utopian potentiality is undermined by the content of the magazine, which reiterates, by contrast, a terminal conflation of equality, as a political objective, with the achieved reality of access to legal marriage. Equality is not imagined as a mobilising vision, or open possibility, but as a punctual event, and as having been definitively achieved in the Irish republic on 22 May 2015. This is reiterated by the reminder that, in this world-view, equality is only open insofar as it was yet, at this point in 2019, to be fully achieved in Northern Ireland.[35]

The tensions inherent to the conception of equality mobilised in the 2015 referendum also come into sharp relief when we juxtapose that referendum with the citizenship referendum in 2004. In 2015, following a higher than usual turnout, 62 per cent of the Irish electorate who cast their ballot voted in favour of marriage equality, extending marriage rights to same-sex couples. In 2004 just under 80 per cent of the Irish electorate who cast their ballot voted to redefine Irish citizenship on grounds of descent or blood rather than place of birth. In short, after the referendum was passed a child born in the state was no longer automatically entitled to Irish citizenship. During the referendum campaign, some politicians, notably the then minister for justice Michael McDowell, had raised an entirely fictitious spectre of Dublin's maternity hospitals being 'flooded' by migrant women, mainly from African countries, giving birth just to acquire citizenship for their children and thus the right of residence for their families. McDowell's scaremongering meant that the transition from a racial to a racist state, to use Ronit Lentin's terms, was explicitly gendered.[36]

In her analysis of the 2004 referendum, Anne Mulhall argues that this confected scenario promoted the idea of 'a vulnerable state under siege from exploitative foreign invaders [which] effectively coded certain women and children as undesirable on grounds of their national origin and ethnic identifications'. Mulhall connected the Irish state's policies of 'racial management' with its ban on abortion, since removed by referendum in 2018, as part of the same bio-political dynamic: 'the racially marked woman as producer of an undesirable future who must therefore be managed by expulsion if necessary is the bio-political complement to the ethnically desirable, presumptively white woman who is, on the other hand, legislatively coerced into reproducing the nation's aspirational future'.[37]

What happens when we juxtapose the referendum results in 2004 and 2015? An optimistic reading would see the 2004 decision as anomalous; an unfortunate, atavistic resurgence of the old nativism that we hoped had been consigned to the past. The 2015 result would then reassure us that political equilibrium has been restored, and that the country is safely back on the historical trajectory of modernisation and liberal pluralism; the sin of 2004 redeemed by the good work of 2015, as it were. However, it is worth recalling that in 2004 a 'yes' vote, in favour of redefining citizenship by descent, was explicitly presented, by McDowell among others, not in traditional nationalist terms but as its opposite: a vote for liberalisation and modernisation, since it would bring Ireland's citizenship laws into closer alignment with the European 'norm'. Unfortunately, then, there is also a more pessimistic interpretation available of the relationship between these two events. Rather than being opposed in meaning, the two referendums present the negative and positive faces of one bio-political dynamic. Each result was one component of the *same* process of redefining who counts as a legitimate citizen; a bio-political dynamic in which, as Mulhall observes, 'legitimation for some inevitably entails de-legitimation for others'.[38]

The year after the 2004 referendum, the organisers of the Dublin Lesbian and Gay Film Festival controversially invited McDowell to open the event. This was a cynical piece of political horse-trading. In return for the minister looking favourably on proposals for enacting civil partnership then before him, an LGBT organisation would give him a media-friendly public platform to burnish his 'socially liberal' credentials at a time when his actual policies – particularly in relation to migrants, refugees and social welfare provision for people with disabilities – were reactionary, illiberal and entirely counter to any conception of equality.

Describing the scene on that evening of the film festival opening in 2005, when those attending walked past members of Ireland's migrant communities protesting outside, Mulhall suggests a startling reversal of roles. In his speech McDowell painted a picture of Dublin as a modern 'successful city' and a space of multiculturalism and diversity; he recruited the city's lesbian and gay community as guarantors of this 'diverse heterogeneous sense of Irish-ness that will replace the narrow self-image of monochrome Catholic nationalist Ireland'.[39] However, the presence of the protesting migrant bodies outside made visible the 'narrow' racist exclusions on which the minister's shallow pluralism and cosmopolitanism silently rested. Insofar as it was they who disrupted, challenged and confronted the status quo, Mulhall argues, 'the agents of "queerness" in this scene are not, then, the largely white, largely middle-class queers in attendance but the heterosexual racialized mothers and their disenfranchised children'.[40] In short then, the broadening of citizenship to include the right to same-sex marriage and the narrowing of citizenship to exclude migrants may not be opposed political developments, one progressive and the other regressive, but inextricably part of the same process. While securing one set of sexual and political rights, progressive social movements can simultaneously contribute to the construction of a neoliberal bio-political regime that denies different rights to others.

Since 2015 there has been considerable continuity between those who advocated for same-sex marriage rights and those supporting the campaign to end the Irish state's direct provision system. *GCN*, for instance, has actively supported this campaign. This is unsurprising. As mobilising slogans such as 'Just Love' and 'Marriage Equality' encapsulated, the demand for marriage rights was predicated on a conception of inalienable human rights, and specifically on demanding the fullest recognition, vindication and protection of those rights; constitutionally by the state but also symbolically by the collective – the 'nation' or 'community'. The denial of their human rights to those who arrived in Ireland seeking asylum only to be incarcerated, for years on end in many cases, in the direct provision apparatus takes a far more visceral, and vicious, form – not merely the wholesale denial of each person's humanity and autonomy, but an active and systematic policy of humiliation and degradation. Clearly the effects of that policy on its victims are different to the effects of being excluded from the institution of legal marriage. Nevertheless, the principle is consistent: the policies of a democratic state must always be predicated on vindicating the rights and dignity of those who stand before it, regardless of their differences (of sexual orientation or national origin or citizenship status).

The difficulty is that the direct provision policy is not only driven by bigotry, racism and xenophobia. Direct provision is also neoliberal ideology in practice; indeed, it is exemplary of that prevailing orthodoxy. By adopting this approach to the asylum application process, the Irish state conformed to the demand that the neoliberal state should be a managerial, not a democratic, entity regulating the contractual outsourcing of its welfare obligations to the market. As Bulelani Mfaco points out, the direct provision system has been extremely lucrative for some. Since the system was established in 2000, the Irish state has given in excess of 1.3 billion euro to the private companies operating this carceral infrastructure. As Mfaco demonstrates in some detail, an alternative system in which the state provided those applying for asylum with public housing, along with the right to either claim regular welfare payments or to seek paid work according to their individual circumstances, would have conformed with human rights norms while also costing far less money.[41] And so, the operation of the system thoroughly undermines that mendacious rhetoric of 'efficiency': magical thinking which inspires such unswerving faith in the illusory superiority of for-profit over public service provision.

Thus, the direct provision system exemplifies the neoliberal state in action. It also exemplifies how, in the dominant ideology, all other criteria of value are subordinate to the profit motive. Consequently, the means of fulfilling our human needs, in all their diversity, is individualised and privatised in conformity with this market logic. Here we can identify a common theme uniting the stories in the *GCN* wedding issue and the stories of survivors of the direct provision system, stories which are otherwise so different in tone.[42] One set of stories illustrates the market striving to commodify and monetise 'happiness'. The other set illustrates the market striving to commodify and monetise vulnerability and despair. Juxtaposing these stories can yield hope, enabling us to perceive the common pattern and grasp the ideological framework underpinning the structure of contemporary class relations – the ideology which dominates 'our' freedom as much as the unfreedom of others. At the same time, taken together these stories also present something more unpalatable. This is the bitter irony confronting those advocates of same-sex marriage rights now supporting the campaign to end direct provision. The contractual rhetoric of equality mobilised for achieving that goal of marriage rights confers an aura of political progressiveness and moral legitimacy over the ideology which underpins the direct provision system.

These contradictions are distilled in the images circulated on digital media platforms by Paul Ryan's respondents, in his study of male sex work in contemporary Dublin. Ryan's interlocutors were young men who had migrated to Dublin, mostly from Brazil and Venezuela, and mostly on student visas. While their legal status is relatively more secure than that of those seeking asylum, and certainly gives them far greater autonomy and freedom, it leaves them financially precarious: large debts after financing their move; exorbitant rents for accommodation in Dublin; limited opportunities for underpaid, highly casualised employment.

Ryan advocates for a harm-reduction approach to sex work; that is, legal and social policies which promote the well-being and safety of those involved in such work. His respondents do not present themselves in that role of a victim passively awaiting rescue promulgated in the neo-abolitionist narrative of 'prostitution', but nor do they conform to the 'happy hooker' trope found in facile libertarian celebrations of sex work as a style of bohemian freedom. As Ryan observes, his respondents 'speak about what they *do*, not about who they *are*'.[43] In short, they think of sex work *as* work. They may feel ambivalent or realistic about this work, but they do not celebrate it or feel victimised. This work is, after all, not intrinsically more or less exploitative than many other forms of labour, especially in the services industry.

This work begins on their bodies. For Ryan's respondents, the gym is a site of community. As several of his Brazilian respondents joked, arranging gym membership is one of the easiest administrative tasks for a new arrival, since so many gym employees speak Portuguese.[44] The gym is also a site of 'aesthetic labour', as Ryan describes it, where the men create the type of body, a lean cisgendered male body armoured in musculature, that is most highly prized, that can be converted into 'physical' and 'erotic' 'capital' in contemporary gay male culture. In their case, that ideal body type is also explicitly racialised. For their Irish clients, these South American men embody, or, more precisely, perform the role of 'an imagined exotic other – brown-eyed, not too pale, but not too dark'. As Ryan notes, this conforms with research from elsewhere on racialised gay identities online, which found that 'participants categorised Latinos as sensual, erotic and passionate … creating parameters with which sex workers constructed their racial identities online'.[45]

In the gym the human body is subjected to what Marcuse identified as the performance principle. In *Eros and Civilisation* (1955) Marcuse challenged Freud's view of repression. Formulated most vividly and tragically in *Civilisation and its Discontents* (1929), Freud saw repression as inevitable in the formation of human subjects and as potentially socially productive since it leads to the sublimation of libidinal drives into other aims such as scientific or artistic innovation. In this view, the sublimation of repressed drives is the indispensable element in the creation of human culture. In Freud's tragic paradox, human culture – 'civilisation' – is essential to preserve human beings from their aggressive drives, and yet submitting to the repressive demands placed on the psyche by that culture inevitably generates profound unhappiness.

While accepting that some repression might be an inevitable element of psychic formation, Marcuse argued that capitalism generated 'surplus repression' through the harnessing of our drives, energies and potentialities into the narrow objective of alienated labour. As Finn Bowring observes, 'the repressiveness of modern civilisation – which for Marcuse is embodied in the puritanical "performance principle" that demands endless toil – is no longer justified by a wild and merciless nature, but is instead perpetuated in the interests of domination. These interests are served by the manufacturing of needs, the hierarchical distribution of scarcity, and the imposition of unnecessary labour'.[46] In sum, the accumulation of surplus value requires surplus repression.

For Marcuse the performance principle is the specific reality principle of modern capitalist society. It describes a distinctive form of unfreedom characteristic of 'an antagonistic and acquisitive society in the process of constant expansion' where 'domination has been increasingly rationalised'. In this society, the majority of people 'while they work do not fulfil their own needs and faculties but work in alienation ... labour time, which is the largest part of the individual's life time, is painful time, for alienated labour is absence of gratification, the negation of the pleasure principle'.[47]

The photos of their shirtless bodies circulated by Ryan's respondents, on Grindr, Instagram and other social media platforms, signify a form of male desirability in which this performance principle is erotically embodied: sculpted bodies as the exchange value extracted from the relentless labour to 'produce' such results. Of course, we do not have to look very far in our culture to realise that erotic enthralment to embodiments of honed, sculpted masculinity extends far beyond gay male culture. For instance, we need look no further than the ubiquity of male team sports in contemporary life. Living under a cultural dominant that constitutively engenders anxiety and precariousness, as we all do, must invariably lead us to form strong libidinal investments in symbols of strength and invulnerability. In our culture, the finely honed – and heavily commodified through advertising and branding – body of the male sports star functions as just such an object of psychic reassurance.

In the gym, the human body is also a site of investment for Ryan's respondents; investing effort now will yield results later. As Wendy Brown argues, the dispersal of economic logic, specifically the logic of finance capital, through everyday life is a defining characteristic of neoliberal political rationality.[48] This does not mean that all aspects of one's life are expected to be directly monetised. But we are expected to conceptualise all aspects of our social and ethical conduct – education, our intimate relationship and so on – through the calculus of cost-benefit analysis, investment and profit-seeking. In this light, viewed as sex *workers*, the men in Ryan's study come to appear not as stigmatised or marginalised but as exemplary. They embody a version of the neoliberal entrepreneurial self – anxiously propelled towards being flexibly resourceful – to which we are all encouraged to aspire.

If the work of sex work begins on the body for these men, it continues with displaying the body and specifically with curating their images on social media. For Ryan's respondents, the evolution of what Jodi Dean termed 'communicative capitalism' has created the opportunity to earn much-needed income.[49] Arguably, in their case, it has created the potential to be much better remunerated, relatively, than in similarly casualised but low-paid work (fast food delivery, for instance). But working with social media for financial gain in this way also demands a high degree of resilience: managing the stress of an unpredictable, precarious income, as well as the demands of a form of 'work' which is indistinguishable from 'leisure', since the curation of their online profiles is unceasing. Again, far from being atypical, their labour exemplifies working conditions more generally in the contemporary 'gig economy'. Promising greater freedom – parasitically extracting positive value from terms like 'choice', 'flexibility' and 'creativity' – neoliberalism explicitly undermines any distinction between 'free time' and 'work time', thereby also undermining the protections for paid labour secured by unionised workers during the twentieth century. Invariably, re-signifying 'work' and 'free' time like this entrenches class divisions – flexibility for the few is anxious precarity for the many.

If the men refuse to define themselves as sex workers but as engaged in sex work, social media platforms have facilitated that distinction. The men avoid designated websites advertising escort services. Instead they creatively and dynamically curate their image on social media platforms to maintain a degree of ambiguity about what precisely is being performed or offered. They are, in Ryan's memorable phrase, 'pop-up escorts'.[50] Of course, this is partly to disguise their engagement in transactional sex and to avoid the stigma associated with sex work, especially in their personal relationships. More crucially though, maintaining that ambiguity is essential to the transaction. Unlike the relatively straightforward exchange of money for the performance of sexual acts advertised on the escort sites, what Ryan's respondents offer to those who give them money or gifts is less easily defined.

What is striking about their stories is the degree to which 'sex work' so often does not actually involve 'sex'. From 'real life', they recount episodes of clients paying them to chat over coffee, or to train with them in the gym or, in one especially poignant anecdote, to simply look at their body and weep.[51] Likewise, in 'digital life' the images – photos, video clips – which they post respond to a variety of emotional needs that are only partially reducible to sexual desire and pleasure. Obviously, some of the images, especially on the Onlyfans platform, are intended to be consumed as porn. However, the majority of the images, especially on Instagram, convey something else: a 'successful' lifestyle that the viewer may desire to live – being manly and sexy in the gym; the glamour of travelling in style to European cities – and, at the same time, an 'ordinary' life – sleepy-eyed and tousle-haired first thing in the morning – that the viewer *feels* like they are sharing. In short, what is being monetised here is not only, or not necessarily, the need for sexual pleasure but a much more amorphous need for human intimacy.[52]

What if we juxtapose the 'Viva School of Dance' ad with these images posted on social media? Here we could easily evoke the concept of individual choice that is so powerfully operative in contemporary culture: some gay men 'choose' to get married, while others 'choose' to pay for sex. The purpose of the 2015 referendum, after all, was to secure a right to marry and not to impose an obligation on everybody to do so. Arguably, the transaction encoded in the online images exemplifies the contractual model of equality which subtended the achievement of marriage rights encoded in the advertising image. This is the neat symmetry of the marketplace. Ryan's respondents have 'physical and erotic capital' and need money; their clients have money and need sexual pleasure and intimacy. Everybody is 'equally' free to consent to the transaction.

But, of course, as the men's stories make perfectly clear, this symmetry is illusory. While they are not the powerless victims of the neo-abolitionist imagination, they are precarious workers navigating a social environment that offers opportunities and hostility in equal measure. They are not powerless, but power is an essential component of these transactions. The men labour strenuously to embody, and perform, a style of 'powerfulness' that is so desirable to their clients. Most obviously the literal embodiment of that powerfulness – muscles on their body – requires arduous physical labour in the gym. At the same time, curating their digital persona – which is just as essential – requires mental and emotional labour that is unceasing and envelops their whole lives. Conversely, while their clients' desire for this illusion of powerfulness appears abject, they nevertheless enjoy a degree of power that comes with money and security (and with being white and male) in our society.

In short, the men's stories offer a condensed and illuminating insight into that complex dynamic relationship between our erotic, emotional and material needs, on one hand, and the radical disparities of power and wealth in late capitalist society, on the other. Their stories undermine the rhetoric of contractual equality central to neoliberal ideology and progressive sexual politics alike. And their stories bring into focus a defining paradox of post-marriage equality Ireland. As *lesbian and gay citizens* many of us now enjoy an expanded freedom to fulfil our emotional and erotic needs. We have, broadly speaking, attained a degree of legal and social equality. But as *citizens* we confront the same challenges as all citizens and residents of this country: an economic and social structure where access to the basic needs of life – most notably healthcare, housing and education – is fundamentally determined by the uneven distribution of wealth. In other words, after marriage equality we are equal citizens in a radically unequal society – one where the achievement of marriage equality grants legitimacy to those structures of inequality.

Vulnerability

Una Mullally's *In the Name of Love* (2014) is formally the most interesting analysis of the campaign for marriage equality in Ireland of those published thus far. For one thing, her book was published in the year before the referendum, so it ends with the outcome as an open possibility. Therefore, the book is a call to mobilise rather than a finished chronicle. More significantly, Mullally chose an oral history format. The book is composed of interviews with seventy-five people, with extracts, of varying lengths, from these interviews spliced together in a recursive pattern so that the book reads like an unfolding conversation. This dialogical style is enhanced by the wide range of her interviewees, and by her care to include a spectrum of competing perspectives, including those ambivalent about the institution of marriage and critics from a radical left-queer-feminist standpoint. Most striking are the voices of those reflecting on the gradual evolution in their own thoughts and feelings. Mullally's multi-perspectival narrative conveys the sense of an evolving and dynamic mobilisation around a political objective. Her style accentuates the 'movement' as form of *move-ment*: a contradictory, contested but democratic process.

This stands in contrast with the monological perspective in subsequent book-length accounts. As the subtitle suggests, *Ireland Says Yes: The inside story of how the vote for marriage equality was won* (2016), by Gráinne Healy, Brian Sheehan and the late Noel Whelan, tells the story from the view of three leading figures in the 'yes' campaign. The book is, as it were, about *how* to mobilise people rather than about capturing the dynamic experience of mobilisation. The narrative perspective reiterates strategy over mobilisation and is therefore hierarchical rather than democratic. The implication is that people are inert matter to be skilfully nudged and formed.

By contrast, the perspective in Sonja Tiernan's *The History of Marriage Equality in Ireland: A social revolution begins* (2020) is not from the 'inside' but the 'outside'. Evidently, Tiernan is profoundly committed, politically and personally, to the campaign for marriage equality. Yet, her style and tone accentuate the 'objectivity' of the expert sociological observer. Not surprisingly then, the narrative likewise prioritises expertise – the voices and actions of lawyers, politicians, journalists and professionalised activists/lobbyists predominate. The titular reference to 'revolution' is therefore perplexing and paradoxical. Taken together, the title and the content suggest that the expedient site of revolution is never the street but the office, the meeting room and the courthouse. In short, that much overworked synecdoche: the 'corridors of power'. And, contrary to Gil Scott-Heron's famous admonition, it appears that the revolution will be televised. Or more accurately, the revolution will be televisual; Tiernan's account heavily emphasises the central role of media strategy. It is also striking that in the title the word 'revolution' needs to be qualified by the word 'social'. This implies that any revolutionary transformation of the economic order is an entirely separate – and from this perspective wholly *unnecessary* – political objective. In this account, 'revolution' appears to be identical with 'reform'.

This singular identification of progress and social change with liberal reformism is reiterated by Tiernan's neatly drawn lines of confrontation. In this heroic political narrative, the only antagonists of marriage equality are conservatives. Ultimately, they are wrong-footed and defeated but only just, so that we must remain vigilant and united against them. In this diminished spectrum of possibilities, any radical political views to the left of the liberal centre simply disappear. For instance, it is notable that the articles by Anne Mulhall and Aidan Beatty, referred to in the 'Equality' section above, are not listed in the extensive bibliography. In this way, any critical perspectives on marriage equality, from a radical/left queer-affirmative rather than conservative position, are not challenged or disputed but simply banished to the realm of the unthinkable. This rigidly linear schema of social change contrasts with the dialectical perspective that emerges in Mullally's narrative, with its conflicting and conflicted positions. In this context, Mullally's and Tiernan's contrasting approaches to one part of the history of marriage equality in Ireland is illuminating. In 2010 the then government published proposed legislation, which had been long in development, to introduce civil partnership in Ireland. This event brought into the open a conflict among Irish LGBT political activists that had been simmering over the preceding years. Essentially this pitched those who had actively sought civil partnership, seeing it as an achievable goal that would improve people's lives, against those who believed that supporting such legislation, rather than campaigning for marriage, was an unconscionable betrayal of the cause of full equality. In Mullally's narrative this significant political debate is explored in considerable detail, with the clash of perspectives capturing its complexity, intensity and occasional bitterness. In Tiernan's account all of this is politely summarised in a few neutrally descriptive paragraphs; in this view, the only dialogue that really counts is never between lesbian and gay activists but with the state.[53]

Mullally begins her account in 1982 and 1983, noting a significant confluence of events in those two years. In April 1983 David Norris' legal action, challenging the constitutionality of the laws criminalising sex between men, was rejected by the Supreme Court. Though two dissenting judges supported Norris, the majority verdict went against him and the chief justice's language was gratuitously offensive in delivering his judgement. Meanwhile during 1982 three gay men – Charles Self, John Roche and Declan Flynn – were murdered in separate incidents in Dublin and Cork. Charles Self was murdered in his own home and his killer was never identified. John Roche was murdered in a Cork hotel room, and Michael O'Connor was found guilty of manslaughter rather than murder. These two killings created a great deal of anxiety in the gay community. This was exacerbated in Dublin by the garda conduct of the investigation into Charles Self's murder, which appeared to prioritise harassing gay men over arresting the murderer.

In September 1982 Declan Flynn was killed when he was attacked by a group of teenagers in Fairview Park. The park was a popular cruising ground, and in the weeks before this attack the group had already attacked about twenty men there. In March 1983 four teenagers were tried for killing Declan Flynn and found guilty but given suspended sentences. Later that day they were welcomed home to their neighbourhood amid scenes of public celebration. In the lesbian and gay community, the deep levels of anger and dismay at this outcome precipitated a protest march, with several hundred participants, through Fairview Park. Facilitated by the organisation of that protest march, the first Gay Pride march in Dublin was held in June of that year.

In her introduction Mullally writes that out of these

events, 'a righteous anger was born' in the gay community. Likewise, she argues that what happened in Fairview Park on 9 September 1982 'changed Irish history'.[54] This is a compelling argument. The brutality of Declan Flynn's murder, and the injustice perpetrated by the court in treating his killers so leniently, was clearly a significant catalyst for the nascent lesbian and gay political movement in Ireland. Mullally's multi-vocal account emphasises how this political mobilisation was dialectical. The political achievement of justice (recognition; rights; protection from discrimination) was precipitated by an act of such terrible injustice. But, as her interviewees reiterate, this was only possible because the political conditions were already in place, after a decade of feminist and lesbian and gay activism, for grief, shock and anger to be reframed and translated into political action and a demand for justice. Declan Flynn's awful fate could only become emblematic of the generalised oppression confronting lesbian and gay men in Ireland more widely because an emergent intellectual and political framework existed to facilitate it becoming so.

Unfortunately, since Mullally's book this narrative of the Irish lesbian and gay rights movement has been simplified in the Irish media. In the first six months of 2020 alone, there were articles about Declan Flynn's death in *GCN*, *Hot Press*, *Image*, and the news websites DublinLive and IrishCentral, along with an RTÉ podcast by the drag performer and activist Panti Bliss (Rory O'Neill). There is an interesting tension between two impulses here.

On one hand, there is a commendable desire to remember, reminding older generations in Irish society of what, for the majority, they tolerated, while providing younger generations with some historical perspective, and particularly helping younger LGBT people to develop some sense of a shared, collective Irish queer history.

At the same time, there is a disquieting fascination with the dead body of a gay man, along with the narrative emphasis on that act of violence as the defining and originary moment of lesbian and gay politics in Ireland. Thus, for instance, the headline in *Hot Press*: 'The Road to Marriage Equality: Remembering Declan Flynn'; to mark the fifth anniversary of the marriage referendum the magazine republished an article first published in 1983.[55] Likewise, *GCN* and *Image*: 'Declan Flynn: The Fairview murder that ignited the Irish pride movement' and 'The Murder of Declan Flynn and the History of Dublin Pride'.[56] In place of Mullally's dialectic, here we get a monocausal, linear model of historical progress. The singular event displaces the dynamic movement, and the freedoms of the present are defined solely in contrast with the oppression of the past. More crucially, the defining impulse propelling political mobilisation is passive victimhood, embodied in Declan Flynn's tragic death as it is now memorialised, rather than any active, revolutionary demand for justice or transformation of the social order.

This prompts two questions. Firstly, how does situating the murder of a gay man so centrally to our conception of progressive sexual politics determine our political vision? In what way does it inform our political demands and shape our historical perspective – not just our perspective on the past but, more urgently, on the future? Secondly, how might we mourn Declan Flynn? Is it possible to mourn him without symbolically reproducing the physical violence that was done to him and reducing the meaning of his life, in all its richness, to the manner of his death?[57]

To begin reflecting on these questions we might turn to Judith Butler, for whom the politics of mourning has been a persistent concern. In 'Violence, Mourning, Politics', Butler argues that, contrary to our common perception of mourning as privatising and apolitical, grief can 'furnish a sense of political community of a complex order'.[58] In reality, Butler suggests, grieving does not follow the neatly linear stages identified in pop psychology but washes over us in sudden and unexpected waves of emotion. We are undone and dispossessed by grief, and are thus made aware, affectively and viscerally, of our fundamental vulnerability and dependence on others. Writing in the wake of the 2001 attacks on New York and Washington, and the subsequent invasions of Afghanistan and Iraq by US-led forces, Butler is aware that this perception of vulnerability can be politicised in very different ways. One such is the transformation of grief into rage: the urge to deny one's vulnerability by violently imposing that condition on others. On the other hand, Butler is also hopeful that 'mindfulness of vulnerability' can become the basis for a different type of politics through which 'we might critically evaluate and oppose the conditions under which certain human lives are more vulnerable than others, and thus certain human lives are more grievable than others'.[59]

Butler's conception of 'vulnerability' stands in contrast with the conception of 'injury' identified by Wendy Brown. In *States of Injury* Brown addressed what she termed the 'problematic of politicised identity'.[60] Her particular focus was on the United States in the 1990s, while also mapping deeper discursive and historical currents underpinning this political dynamic in late capitalism. Brown alerts us to a central paradox here: forms of politicised identity underpinned various movements for progressive social change in the late twentieth century (anti-imperialism; anti-racism; liberal feminism; LGBT rights), yet politicised identity invariably reinforces the existing ideological and social structures of capitalist liberal democracy. This paradox stems from the political grammar and the type of demands formulated in the name of politicised identities. In their most essential form those demands centre on recognition and inclusion. But, and here is a second paradox, while ostensibly securing redress and justice, the demand for recognition institutionalises and entrenches the same discursive, social and psychic processes of subjection and injury through which stigmatised identities are formed. Thus, for instance, in exchange for legal protection from homophobic discrimination, lesbian and gay people must symbolically conform to the idea that such homophobia cannot be transcended since their identity is structured around always being a potential victim of homophobia. Rather than freedom, what is achieved is a permutation or recalibration within the existing forms of regulation and reification.

These demands for recognition and inclusion are propelled by a conception of identity predicated on injury. In this way, Brown argues, politicised identity must be understood as caused by, and reaction against, a pervasive *ressentiment* – the fusion of powerlessness, abjection and anger which Nietzsche identified as intrinsic to modernity. The cultural ubiquity of injury, as an identity-defining affect, is symptomatic of the contradictions each of us faces in late capitalism. On one side, we confront a capitalist world system where our lives are determined by de-territorialised and potentially cataclysmic process-es that are difficult to apprehend let alone bring under democratic control: financialisation; outsourced product-ion; ecological destruction and climate change. On the other, neoliberal political rationality imposes a relentless expectation that we exercise rigorous control over our fate while constructing well-managed lives as model entrepreneurial subjects. This Brown describes as a society 'in which individuals are buffeted and controlled by global configurations of disciplinary and capitalist power of extraordinary proportions, and are at the same time nakedly individuated, stripped of reprieve from relentless exposure and accountability for themselves'.[61]

In a third paradox, politicised identity is a formation generated in reaction to the oppressive and alienating conditions of capitalism, which at the same time supresses the potential for anti-capitalist critique and politics. In this minoritarian discourse those 'differences' which in reality are an effect of the exploitative structural relations inherent within capitalism are neutralised as attributes inhering in individuals. Any injustice suffered because of these 'differences' can be resolved by individuals aggregating into minority groups. The specific 'interests' of those minority groups can be adjudicated on, and protected by, a supposedly neutral liberal state which is held to be autonomous from capitalism.

Politicised identity re-scripts capitalism's endemic alienation as a question of inclusion and exclusion. Ironically, identity politics finds itself committed to the perpetuation of exclusion, since its political demands are so thoroughly structured by this distinction. As Brown argues, the discourse of inclusion/exclusion presupposes something from which one is excluded that one values and desires since one is seeking inclusion within it. We have already noted this paradox in relation to the campaign for marriage equality: to seek inclusion within the existing institution of marriage is to commit to the continuing exclusion – from the material, legal and symbolic advantages of that institution – of those who are unmarried. If legal marriage were not definitionally exclusive, there would be no motivation for seeking inclusion within it. However, Brown's critique presents a more fundamental challenge to the basis of critical politicised identities. The commitment to the discourse of inclusion/exclusion, she argues, discloses an unacknowledged investment in a 'universal' subjectivity from which 'minorities' are excluded. But in patriarchal and capitalist society this valorised and normative form of subjectivity is, in fact, not universal at all but is, ironically, itself a 'minority': white, middle-class, heterosexual and masculinist.

Needless to say, Brown clearly distinguishes her critique of politicised identity from the reactionary rejection of identity politics by the political right, which is essentially a vehicle for rearticulating racist, misogynistic, homophobic or transphobic prejudices. Crucially, the logic of politicised identity analysed by Brown is not confined to liberal, progressive or radical movements. Notwithstanding its rejection of 'identity politics', right-wing politics is in fact discursively organised around various formulations of national, ethnic, religious and gendered identity and impelled by deep reservoirs of *ressentiment*. Over two decades after Brown was writing, politics almost everywhere is even more unrelentingly and violently dominated by reactionary, right-wing forms of politicised identity: religious fundamentalism; ethno-nationalism; white supremacy; 'inceldom'.

Of course, as Judith Butler reminds us, progressive forms of identity politics are still strategically indispensable and powerfully operative for the feminist and lesbian/gay social movements, as for the political mobilisation of minorities defined by race, disability, ethnicity and sex/gender in the Western democracies and globally. It is politically essential to demand bodily integrity and self-determination, and to use the language of individual autonomy, to secure legal protections and entitlements. In the Irish context the successful feminist-led campaign to repeal the constitutional ban on abortion, culminating in the 2018 referendum, is the most notable recent demonstration of the efficacy of mobilising around such claims.[62]

Butler does not argue for an end to such politics, but she challenges us to simultaneously imagine a different form of politics. She challenges us to open up 'another kind of normative aspiration within the field of politics ... if I am struggling for autonomy, do I not need to be struggling for something else as well, a conception of myself as invariably in community, impressed upon by others, impinging on them as well in ways that are not fully in my control or clearly predictable'.[63]

Centrally this form of politics which Butler calls for would not be premised on the autonomy and identity of the sovereign subject but on the condition of vulnerability intrinsic to the human body. As Butler observes, 'the body implies mortality, vulnerability, agency: the skin and the flesh expose us to the gaze of others, but also to touch, and to violence, and bodies put us at risk of becoming the agency and instrument of all these as well. Although we struggle for rights over our own bodies, the bodies for which we struggle are not quite ever only our own'.[64] Confronting our bodily vulnerability is a visceral reminder that 'we are all born in a position of radical dependency'.[65] Moreover it is not that we overcome or move beyond that radical dependency as we grow and develop. In every moment of our lives, we only survive because the resources necessary to sustain human life, and to create the conditions for human flourishing, are made available to us by the ecosystem we inhabit and by the labour and love of other humans. It is not only that we are more dependent when newly born or aged, but also that the moments of our birth and our death are the most clarifying reminders of the vulnerability and dependency which we *always* inhabit.

This encounter with the material reality of our interdependence is a powerful solvent of the ideology of bourgeois individualism, since the disavowal of interdependence is essential to that ideology. As Butler puts it, 'we have become creatures who constantly imagine a self-sufficiency, only to find that image of ourselves undermined repeatedly in the course of life'.[66] To mobilise politically around human interdependence requires conceptualising our consciousness and sense of self as relational rather than separative. But not relational in the conventional aggregative understanding of relationality as two autonomous selves entering into relationship with each other. In other words, not 'I' relating to 'you', but the profoundly unsettling realisation that there is in fact no 'I' prior to, or independent of, that relationship with 'you'.[67] This Butler describes as 'another way of imagining community ... which affirms relationality not only as a descriptive or historical fact of our formation, but also as an ongoing normative dimension of our social and political lives, one in which we are compelled to take stock of our interdependence'.[68]

To recognise vulnerability as ontological, as intrinsic to human existence as such, is also, as Butler reminds us, to recognise vulnerability as political. In the capitalist world-system the distribution of corporeal vulnerability – degrees of exposure to violence, exploitation and want – is, to put it mildly, obscenely inequitable. And to recognise that we are radically dependent on the world's resources and on the labour of others is to confront how, in our current system, the extraction of those resources is often recklessly destructive, and that labour is invariably alienated and punitively exploited. To figure the human body as vulnerable is therefore to figure that body dialectically. Vulnerability is the visceral mark of capitalist exploitation, but also the visceral source of potential revolt against it.

The tension between these contrasting political-affective potentialities – injury and vulnerability – was vividly illuminated in contemporary Irish culture in *Faultline*, a theatre production by the Dublin-based company ANU, in conjunction with the Gate Theatre, in autumn and winter 2019. As with ANU's other productions, this was a site-specific performance which took place in the basement of a Georgian building on Dublin's Parnell Square. In the 1970s the Irish Gay

Rights Movement had its offices, and ran a nightclub for its members, in a building on the opposite side of the square. And as with those other productions, the style of performance was immersive. The audience – restricted in number for each show – moved through a series of spaces (a dance floor and bar; public bathroom; the offices from which a telephone helpline was being run) encountering a different performance in each space. As an audience member, the order in which you encountered the performances depended on which of two groups you were randomly assigned to when first entering the space.

The extensive use of carefully curated detail in the set design established the time period in the early 1980s. However, an audience member remained heavily dependent on the company's description of the production, which they would have read in advance, to orientate themselves. According to this information, the production was developed from source materials in the Irish Queer Archive (now held in the National Library of Ireland) about the effects of the three killings in 1982, and the garda investigation into the killing of Charles Self, on the lesbian and gay community in Dublin. In the actual performances though this historical context was only alluded to with any degree of specificity in one episode, that in the 'helpline office'.

ANU's brief manifesto about the production offered a highly specific interpretation of the archival material. This presented as historical fact the idea of an organised pogrom by 'Church and State' directed against the lesbian and gay community, which resulted in a 'mass exodus' from Ireland. This account emphasised passive victimhood, effacing entirely the political mobilisation catalysed by these events. Likewise, it effaced the ideological fractures, between liberal assimilationist and Marxist/republican liberationist currents, which those events exacerbated in the Irish lesbian and gay movement; we will return to examine those divergent currents later. Moreover, this interpretation reiterated a rigidly minoritarian conception of Irish lesbians and gay men by distinguishing their emigration as wholly distinct from, rather than on a spectrum with, the many other Irish people of their generation who emigrated in the 1980s. Their 'exodus' – the biblical language, evoking analogies with Jewish historical experience, is striking – was in search of 'anonymity and refuge' – economic necessity, jobs and career opportunities (or indeed the quest for excitement) playing no part in their decision (or lack of). Paradoxically, for a company dedicated to mobilising a radical form of theatre practice to politicise its audience, the implied injunction here is remarkably acquiescent to the status quo: be grateful for what you have now because look at just how unrelentingly terrible it was then.[69]

Strikingly, the political effects of this manifesto were alternatively affirmed and subverted by different parts, or episodes, of the actual production. Two monologues by the cabaret singer Donna Marie (Nandi Bhebe) aestheticised the politics of injury. One was delivered as a 'chat' with the audience while on her smoke break; the other as a viscerally anguished performance 'on stage' in the bar. Crucially, in this narrative of a young woman, who does not seem to identify as lesbian, seeking refuge from racism and marginalisation in a space otherwise occupied by gay men, the historical meaning and specificity of lesbian and gay subcultural/activist spaces is re-signified. Mobilisation, creativity, searching for pleasure and intimacy – all are effaced, and substituted with an amorphously de-politicised vision of a space where temporary shelter, but no claim for redress, is sought by those united only by the experience of injury.

Paradoxically, the aesthetics of immersive theatre, aiming for a transformative encounter between audience and performer, inadvertently contributed to creating the opposite effect – a depoliticising affirmation of the individual over the collective. Aiming to be radically dialogic – performers drawing the audience into conversation – the effect was more a simulacrum of intimacy. Arguably, the effect was actually less dialogic than the experience in 'traditional' theatre practice of watching from a distance as actors enact competing viewpoints on a stage. As Brecht famously argued, experimental and stylised, deliberately 'theatrical' stage productions can, by 'alienating' the audience, potentially generate clarifying moments of recognition; sudden insights into ideological contradiction and into our historical conditions. By contrast, by immersing us so completely in the actuality of a strenuously realised 'reality' – a 'reality' with a solidity that comes to feel impossible to shift – immersive and site-specific theatre practice loses the potential for such discombobulating moments of recognition. At worst, the strongest affect is awkwardness and embarrassment; at best, as in *Faultline*, it is a wholly emotional *identification* with the character that is drained of any historical or political dimension.

Nevertheless, two episodes in the production generated more dynamic political affects. Importantly, the history of lesbian and gay political mobilisation, ignored in the manifesto, featured in the production. In the 'helpline office' Paul (Matthew Malone) was an activist on the point of exhaustion, and his monologue dwelt on this sense of being overwhelmed by the oppressive pressure of unfolding events (Self and Flynn killings; garda investigation into the former) while striving to help others. However, his monologue was preceded by some comic business with the ringing phones, along with an animated conversation with his colleague about how the activists working for the lesbian and gay community should respond to garda harassment. Thus, the dominant mood of the production, with its pervasive emphasis on suffering and victimhood, was challenged in this episode by a more variegated tone conveying a livelier sense of collective mobilisation, political debate and cooperation.

The dominant tone, already established by the manifesto, was similarly disrupted by a dance performance by Matthew Williamson and Stephen Quinn.

This episode, without dialogue or music, took place in the 'club bathroom' – a space in which the ambivalent cultural relationship between 'public' and 'private', such a key faultline in the regulation of male same-sex desire during the twentieth century, is literalised. It began as two solo performances, in which Williamson and Quinn contorted their bodies in a syncopated sequence of percussive, jagged gestures: the body subjected to aggression – twisted, hurled against hard surfaces – but also the body as instrument of aggression. But the body as beautiful and desirable too, in its ragged vulnerability, as the solo performances evolved into a duet which aestheticised the stylised gestures of anonymous cruising – a repertoire once familiar to most gay men, but now presumably consigned to the analogue past – to create an encounter of two male bodies in which violence and intimacy, pleasure and pain, merged.

Framed by the production manifesto, this dance performance could be understood as giving aesthetic expression to the experience of shame. In this reading, the audience were expected to interpret the dancer's bodily contortions as expressing anguish and self-loathing, physical symptoms of a psychic condition that was in turn the effect of a historical condition – living in an oppressive, homophobic society. However, there are two interesting complications worth considering here. One is the potential for a theatre production so obviously motivated by a strongly gay-affirmative and anti-homophobic politics to find itself affirming a sacramentalism which bears the imprint of homophobia. In other words, the audience's expected political affect – recognising the aestheticised bodily expression of anguish and shame as such – depends on the expectation that the audience will recognise cruising as intrinsically disordered, as a dehumanising practice now happily made archaic by gay marriage.

The second is the potential for the human body – the visceral affects on the audience of close proximity to these two bodies in agitated, but also erotic, motion – to undermine and disrupt the aesthetic and political hermeneutic of identity. Put most simply, Williamson's and Quinn's performance affirmed that the defining bodily experience of being a gay man might not actually be psychic injury after all but sharing sexual pleasure, in all its varied forms, and intimacy with another man. At first glance that may seem banal and obvious, but in contemporary culture it is surprisingly rare to find that idea articulated. This is almost certainly an effect of the compact underpinning the achievement of marriage equality. The price of recognition is allegiance to a diversified form of homosacramentalism, in which we affirm that sex really is sinful ('unhealthy' in secular parlance) if not redeemed by the marital contract. The desexualisation of gay experience echoes through the performance of self-disclosure demanded by the confessional culture of social media. Thus, it is routine for younger gay men to narrate their life experiences so that the rite of passage defining their 'sexuality' has, it turns out, nothing to do with sex, and their bodies, but is instead composed of the discursive act of 'coming out'.

It is in this context then that we might reflect again on how we remember Declan Flynn and his terrible death. The choice is not between remembering or forgetting this death but between different ways of mourning this man. On one side are those forms of memorialisation in which his death becomes emblematic of a more generalised condition of injury, in which he embodies a psychic condition of injury informing our cultural conception of gay and queer identities as such, and that conception of injury then underpinning a minoritarian politics of redress, recognition and reform. On the other side is the possibility of mourning his death as an encounter with our shared condition of corporeal vulnerability and dependence, that encounter in turn prompting us towards a form of political consciousness predicated on relationality rather than on identity, while also reorienting our political imagination from reform and towards revolution.

Revolution

It is gone from the hill and the glen –
The strong speech of our sires;
It is sunk in the mire and the fen
Of our nameless desires;
We have bartered the speech of the Gael
For a tongue that would pay,
And we stand with the lips of us pale
And all bloodless today;[70]

Despite its ornate diction, this is an extract from a poem which labours under a prosaic title: 'The Irish Language'. It was written by Roger Casement and sent to an acquaintance in 1904 but not published in his lifetime. Here Casement articulates concerns about the rapid decline of the Irish language during the nineteenth century that were expressed more fully elsewhere in Irish political discourse at the time, most notably in Douglas Hyde's 1892 lecture 'On the Necessity of De-Anglicising Ireland'. Earlier in the nineteenth century, mainstream nationalism, led by Daniel O'Connell, took a more sanguine view of the transition from the Irish language to the English language, regarding it as a necessary function of modernisation.[71] In an interesting way, Casement's poem simultaneously looks back, to a time before modern nationalist thought, and forward, beyond its own time into the later twentieth century. In this, the poem is a minor instance of a temporal instability characteristic of his writing more generally, an instability which can be read politically as expressing his rejection of just the type of historical narrative underpinning certain nationalist, as much as imperialist, conceptions of progress.[72]

Casement uses a trope from Gaelic language poetry of the seventeenth and eighteenth century, in which the poet despairs at the decline of the old Gaelic order and the advance of the Anglophone, Protestant order consolidated by the post-Cromwellian settlement. The real anger in this poetry was often directed at the representatives of the Gaelic order for their weakness, and for allowing themselves to be defeated spiritually as much as militarily.[73] Thus, in Casement's poem, it is 'we', not 'they', who are most culpable for bartering 'the speech of the Gael / for a tongue that would pay'. The repudiation of commerce strikes a note that is familiar from the writings of Casement's contemporary cultural nationalists, notably Yeats, playing off the ideas of Matthew Arnold: the loquacious, spontaneous Celt contrasted with Saxon subservience to a sterile contractualism.

Nevertheless, this rejection of instrumentalism can also be read, within the larger context of Casement's intellectual and political career, as indexing his searching indictment of the capitalist ideology underpinning the exploitative global economic order – investigating the devastation unleashed by that system was central to his life's work.

While echoing, or ventriloquising (and, ironically enough, rendering into English), that archaic Gaelic tradition, Casement also turns away from the empiricism underpinning the O'Connellite response to language loss – language is a system of communication, and you can easily switch from one to another – and gestures forward into the twentieth century towards something like the Sapir–Whorf language-thought model (the structure of a language shapes its speakers' world-view) or those ideas about language and cultural identity we associate with George Steiner – language not so much a mode of communication as a structure for creating meaning; a set of emotional, psychic and cultural co-ordinates through which one locates one's identity as an individual and as a member of a community. What happens then when a language becomes historically obsolete – what does this do to the psyche of the individuals and that community? As Hugh observes in Brian Friel's play *Translations* (1980), 'it can happen that a civilisation can be imprisoned in a linguistic contour which no longer matches the landscape of ... fact'.[74] Hence, in Casement's poem, the 'desires' which took shape through the 'strong speech of our sires' have not disappeared with the disappearance of that language, but nor can they be translated into this new language either. They persist, but in this strange, ghostly form as that which is 'nameless' or taboo, and this is reiterated by the spectral image of pale, bloodless lips.

But if the poem seems to gesture forward to these later conceptions of language and identity, it is also very much a nineteenth-century poem in its gendered conception of national identity as an oedipal drama of paternity, manliness and degeneration. Yet, in the midst of all the butch, hyper-reproductive rhetoric of sires and sons, one's ear is caught by that curious phrase: 'our nameless desires'. This must be at least in part due to the echo it carries of another, more scandalous, phrase from those decades: 'the love that dare not speak its name'. While that phrase originated in a poem by Alfred Douglas, it is now most vividly and poignantly associated with another Irishman standing at the bar of British imperial justice, as Casement would do in 1916: Oscar Wilde.

Reflecting on those erotic undertones to Casement's language politics prompts us to think about the relationship between two forms of desire: homoerotic and revolutionary. A useful starting point here is James Penney's distinction between sexual politics and sexualising the political. Sexual politics takes that matrix of gendered and sexual identities produced in determinate historical conditions as the basis of a demand for recognition and as its ultimate horizon. One does not have to look far in our contemporary world to apprehend the continuing necessity and urgency of this project. Nevertheless, as Penney argues, this does not preclude an alternative critical project: understanding how all politics is inherently sexual and exploring 'the libidinal logic, the unconscious fantasies that buttress particular political judgements and desires'.[75] Later we will discuss Ernst Bloch's argument that hope, understood as a fusion of the affective and cognitive, is the indispensable condition for the utopian imagination; here we might just note that desire, like hope, is the ambient state of all transformative politics.

As is well known, Casement produced official reports for the British Foreign Office on conditions in the Belgian Congo (1904) and in the Putumayo region of Amazonia in South America (1911). These were two of the major areas of rubber extraction at the time, and Casement investigated the enslavement and exploitation of the native populations by the rubber industry in both places. What made his reports so compelling was Casement's development of a systematic critique of imperialism, as a global network of exploitative capitalist relations, in which the discursive or textual body is central. Casement's writing exemplifies a powerful interpretive mode in which epistemology and political analysis are affectively grounded. Alongside his notes and drafts for these official reports, Casement was also keeping a private diary. Between his trial and execution, in the summer of 1916, sexually explicit extracts from these were circulated among Casement's influential supporters by agents of the British state with the intention of supressing a campaign for leniency.

Strikingly, Casement uses the constrained and potentially sterile idiom of bureaucratic discourse to generate visceral accounts of malnourished and mutilated bodies, broken by slave labour, torture and disease. By contrast, in the private diary, bodies, and specifically the bodies of men, are a site of pleasure and delight. In a recurring pattern, the desirable male body is a source of visual pleasure to the cruising eye, and despite their terseness, his accounts of sex frequently describe an exchange of pleasure and joy that is surprisingly lyrical. Reading these contrasting accounts of the human body in various states of pain and pleasure, we can see the contradictions of capitalist modernity taking affective form on the human body and in ways of writing about the body.

Angus Mitchell argues that Casement's official writings 'left on the record evidence of an immeasurable, interlinking ethnocide, driven by the insatiable demand for rubber and a financial system unregulated by any sense of moral responsibility to either humanity or the living environment ... when analysed together, his investigations of the transatlantic rubber trade had laid bare the destructive capacity of venture capital and the violently oppressive force of colonial power'.[76] The challenge confronting Casement was to render visible and concrete those abstract and occluded webs of interconnectedness spun by the expanding capitalist world

economy; to tackle 'capitalism's innate tendency to abstract in order to extract', as Rob Nixon describes it in a
different context.[77]

In Nixon's study of contemporary writer-activists who
use their writing to oppose environmental devastation,
he argues that movements for environmental justice
confront twin problems of apprehension and representation. The scale, pace and elongated trajectory of
environmental degradation is difficult to assimilate to
our habitual temporalities of biological and generational
time. This is exacerbated by the somatic and psychic
accelerations of late capitalism, neoliberalism's favoured
model of technocratic politics – focused on immediate
'problems' to be 'solved' not historical processes and
structures – along with unceasing demands on our
attention by communicative capitalism. Moreover, the
effects of environmental destruction are usually displaced
geographically, to spaces distant from those inhabited by
the wealthy and powerful, and socially on to the bodies of
the poor. In addition, the poisonous somatic and cellular
effects of ecological degradation are often literarily
invisible since these are internalised in bodies; and again,
most often in the bodies of the poor. Nixon develops a
distinction between violence as conventionally figured
in political and media discourse – an immediately
apprehensible and spectacular but contained event –
and what he terms the 'slow violence' characteristic of
capitalism. This is violence 'that occurs gradually and
out of sight, a violence of delayed destruction that is

dispersed across space and time, an attritional violence that is typically not viewed as violence at all'.[78] Since it is not spectacular or instantaneous, but 'incremental and accretive, its calamitous repercussions played out across a range of temporal scales', slow violence presents particular narrative and representational challenges. For this reason, Nixon argues that writing can be politically operative since it can 'challenge perceptual habits that downplay the damage slow violence inflicts and bring into imaginative focus apprehensions that elude sensory corroboration'.[79]

Casement begins his 1904 report with his arrival at Léopoldville, the main centre of Belgium's colonial operations in the Congo. As the place-name reiterates, at this point the Congo was not actually administered as a colony but as the personal fiefdom of the Belgian monarch. Casement's account of the settlement there includes visiting a building which he pointedly calls 'an establishment designed as a native hospital':

When I visited the three mud huts which serve the purpose of the native hospital, all of them dilapidated, and two with the thatched roofs almost gone, I found seventeen sleeping sickness patients, male and female, lying about in the utmost dirt. Most of them were lying on the bare ground – several out on the pathway in front of the houses, and one, a woman, had fallen into the fire just prior to my arrival (while in the final insensible stages of the disease) and had burned herself very badly. She had since been well-bandaged, but was still lying out on the ground with her head almost in the fire, and while I sought to speak to her, in turning she upset a pot of scalding water over her shoulder. All the seventeen people I saw were near their end, and on my second visit two days later, the 19th June, I found one of them lying dead out in the open.

In somewhat striking contrast to the neglected state of these people, I found, within a couple of hundred yards of them, the Government workshop for repairing and fitting the steamers. Here all was brightness, care, order, and activity, and it was impossible not to admire and commend the industry which had created and maintained in constant working order this useful establishment.[80]

This description of the human body in distress and pain – particularly the dying woman helplessly injuring herself – is part of a recurring pattern in Casement's writing. Under Leopold's administration, soldiers in the Congo had to account for their use of bullets by providing a severed hand from each corpse they shot while enforcing the rubber-collecting regime; that is, those they shot for refusing to collect rubber, including the population of whole villages as a warning to their neighbours, or those who failed to collect their 'quota'. But in practice the soldiers also severed the hands of the living, in what, as Adam Hochschild argues, was a deliberate policy of terror condoned by senior Belgian officials.[81] Thus Casement's 1904 report contains repeated accounts of bodies left mutilated and disfigured by this practice, such as his description of 'a young man, both of whose hands had been beaten off with the end of rifles against a tree' and 'a young lad of 11 or 12 years of age, whose right hand was cut off at the wrist'.[82] As Séamas Ó Síocháin and Michael O'Sullivan note about the 1904 report, one of its compelling and innovative features was Casement's use of appendixes, 'Inclosures' in his terminology, to ensure that the voices of Africans are given direct expression.[83] One of these is the statement of Mola Ekulite describing the loss of his two hands. Along with a group of other men, he was left tied up overnight and heavy rain caused the ropes binding his wrists to contract. On the following morning, seeing that his swollen hands had been rendered useless by the severity with which the ropes cut into his flesh, the soldiers beat off his hands with rifles. Flogging was another widely used tactic to punish and terrorise the native populations pressed into rubber collection in both the African and South American extractive economies. For this reason, Casement's writing includes recurring descriptions of the scarring left on bodies by this practice: 'of seven men here on the station, three bore obvious broad weals, deep-dyed across their buttocks and thighs ... the marks are deep, and yet everyone takes it as a matter of course'; 'the man's bare buttocks, thighs, and even lower back and loins were severely marked with lashes ... all bore marks of flogging, marks that will not disappear'.[84]

Like the mutilated limbs of the Congolese, these 'indelible marks of the lash' and 'highly instructive backsides', as Casement describes it, offered a visceral indictment of the deliberate use of violence, as a matter of policy, as part of a system of slave labour predicated on extracting profit through terror.[85] By contrast, the sleeping sickness patients described above are dying through neglect and negligence. They are being passively allowed to die in pain rather than being actively brutalised. Yet such wilful neglect can equally serve as an instrument of terror. The message powerfully conveyed by such negligence is that 'native bodies' are merely tools for collecting rubber; beyond that they are useless, worthless and disposable – worth so much less than the well-cared-for riverboats in the adjacent workshop. That message is conveyed most traumatically by the description of a human body left lying around like so much refuse; breaching that most fundamental taboo – the injunction to bury the dead.

Casement's account deliberately juxtaposes the hospital where bodies are carelessly abandoned with the workshop where machines are carefully maintained. This reiterates how the textual body in pain can serve as a representational strategy to overcome the difficulty of apprehending slow violence as a function of the dynamics of global capitalism. The instrumental reasoning that negligently discards unprofitable bodies is inseparable from the entrepreneurial spirit of innovation and adventure that produced the 'excellently constructed' railway that Casement admires a few pages earlier and the fleet of steamships that busily ply their profitable trade on the river. Moreover, his emphasis on describing these modes of transport reiterates the incongruent juxtaposition of temporalities: the technologies of movement and speed alongside the slow pace of bodily immobilisation, decline and death (his observation of how little, apart from one death, changes between his visits). Thus, this episode metonymically reiterates Casement's more general scrambling of the historical narrative underpinning capitalist modernity, with its confident opposition of 'backwardness' and 'progress'. The atrocities Casement uncovered in the Congo and Putumayo were not vestigial, the anomalous survivals of archaic, unenlightened practices, but were a product of modernity. And as the excited rhythm of his prose in the second paragraph conveys – 'all was brightness, care, order, and activity' – even when surrounded by the horror it had wrought, Casement, no more than the rest of us, could not help being moved by this evidence of capitalism's creative energy and vigour.

That Casement was acutely aware of this dialectic of progress and catastrophe – even while it inevitably determined his ideological horizons – is equally apparent in his writing about the body as a site of pleasure. In the 1903 private diary there is a particular concentration of sexual encounters during the three-week holiday Casement spent on Madeira in the spring of that year, while on his way back to Africa to begin his investigations. We can notice a few features in his writing about these encounters. One is his occasional use of phrases in a crude version of Kikongo, the Bantu language of the Congo basin, when he wants to record some more explicitly erotic details.[86] In this way the evocation of these scenes of bodily pleasures taking place thousands of miles from the Congo is haunted by those scenes of bodily pain and trauma recorded elsewhere in Casement's writing because of this linguistic disruption into the flow of the prose and the particular look and sound of these words for the Anglophone reader. Secondly, his cruising and his sexual encounters become part of the rhythm of Casement's daily routine while on the island. The other recurring feature of that pattern is his almost daily visits to the casino. In the diaries the two are very often combined – he will spend the evening at the casino and later spend some time cruising on the walk back to his hotel.[87] The pleasures of gambling and of cruising are very similar: the thrilling excitement of uncertainty, speculation and risk (the risk of losing one's money; the risk of being rejected – or worse); the chance of how the roulette ball may randomly fall; the chance of how the speculative glance or gesture may be received.

In the diaries gambling and cruising are also connected by Casement's daily financial accounting. The diary records his wins and losses at the roulette wheel, along with the money, cigarettes and drink he distributes to lovers: 'Augustinho – Kissed many times. 4 dollars. To Casino, lost £3'.[88] Casement's narration of his sexual encounters implicitly but powerfully protests and repudiates the exploitation and the horror he was investigating, as well as offering escape and relief from it. Nevertheless, some of the same logic underpinning that system of exploitation simultaneously seeps into these private accounts. We might note the obsessive recording and comparing of penis size, the recurring, paradoxical references to 'beautiful types' and his meticulous accounting of money spent, either directly on payments to young men or on dinners, hotel rooms and the like. In this instrumental approach to human relations, the logic which commodifies and exploits the human body as a machine for extracting profit leaves a curious imprint in the diaries as a commodification of other bodies for the extraction of pleasure. As Alan Sinfield observes, in another context, 'our sexual imaginaries probably are informed by hierarchies that are ultimately oppressive, but we have to negotiate within, through and beyond that insight'.[89] Thus the male body, as it is written in Casement's diaries, is at once a utopian space of affective possibilities, promising a richer, humane alternative to the ruthless, instrumental logic of capitalism, while simultaneously reiterating the extraordinary difficulty of imagining such utopian alternatives from within the social relations and historicist epistemology of capitalism.

In April 1910 Casement paid a short visit to Dublin, while on leave from his post as British consul-general in Rio de Janeiro and before he returned to South America with the commission to undertake his Putumayo investigations. On 20 April he records sending a postcard from Dublin Zoo to Ramon.[90] A few pages earlier Ramon is Casement's sexual partner on several occasions during his visit to Buenos Aires; the city's zoo was their regular meeting place. Again, we might note the curious fusion of commercial transaction – 'Ramon 7$000. 10" at least. X' – with the intimacy implied by the shared joke of the postcard.[91] The next day he is back in the Phoenix Park (where Dublin Zoo is located): 'In Phoenix Park, & lovely – at X where F. Cavendish killed.' Here Casement's writing about his sexual encounters generates a distinctive spatial and temporal structure of feeling. The diaries plot an affective map – comprising locations of sexual encounters, as well as locations of memory and fantasy where he recalls other encounters – linking Dublin with Buenos Aires with Rio de Janeiro with Lisbon with Madeira, and so on. This global web of erotic and affective connections shadows the global web generated by the new transport and communication technologies – Casement criss-crossing the Atlantic and the Irish Sea; the postcard making its way to Ramon – but also, of course, the global movements of capital and resources (and of new military technology) underpinning the horrors of rubber extraction in the Congo and Putumayo. Casement also notes that his sexual encounter takes place where two senior figures in the British administration in Ireland, Lord Frederick Cavendish, chief secretary, and Thomas Burke, head of the civil service, had been assassinated by militant Irish nationalists in 1882. Thus, the momentary time of sexual pleasure is woven through the generational and national time of historical events – connected together through the *lieu de mémoire* of the park – just as Casement's commitment to Irish anti-colonial nationalism was woven through his internationalist humanitarian commitments and his analysis of capitalism.[92]

Since the 1990s Casement has been the favourite Irish revolutionary for two generations of Irish intellectuals uneasy with the idea of revolution. The volume of scholarly publications – biographies; annotated editions of his diaries; collections of essays; journal special issues – and popular journalism (including radio and television documentaries) devoted to Casement far exceeds that on other Rising leaders, including prominent figures such as Connolly and Pearse. Of the revolutionary generation Casement has also been particularly fascinating to artists. Within a few months in 2016, for instance, he was the subject of two visual artworks installed in major public galleries, a dance production and a work of contemporary music.[93]

Predictably, the political valences of such commemorative attention vary widely. His biographers, most notably Angus Mitchell and Séamas Ó Síocháin, along with historians such as Adam Hochschild, Margaret O'Callaghan and the late Michael O'Sullivan, are attracted to Casement's radical anti-capitalist and anti-imperialist commitments, his internationalist vision and his civic republicanism. Conversely, Casement's legacy has also been recruited to bolster the legitimacy of the

Irish state and its adherence to neoliberal orthodoxies. Thus, Martin Mansergh's observation that 'the more idealistic side of Irish foreign policy ... followed a straight line from Casement to Mary Robinson'.[94] In passing, we might note the irony that Mansergh was an adviser and subsequently a junior minister in a number of Fianna Fáil-led governments whose actual policies were on the rather less 'idealistic' side of that history: the deliberate reduction of the rights offered to asylum seekers by the 1996 Refugee Act; maintaining a position of 'neutrality' at the United Nations in the face of the Anglo-American neo-imperialist drive to war in 2003, while simultaneously making Irish airport facilities available to US military during the war; the enthusiastic embrace of free market economics and a clear intention to position the Irish elite with the powerful and against the powerless and dispossessed in the global order. In a bitter irony, Casement's memory was marshalled to legitimise the ideological underpinnings of the neoliberal variant on the imperial global order he had opposed.

Reformulating Casement's early-twentieth-century revolutionary anti-capitalist perspective as some form of early-twenty-first-century 'ethical' commitment to neoliberal diversity and pluralism was not confined to conservative politicians. It has also been a recurring feature of the interpretive attention paid to Casement's evident attraction to men, and his erotic life, as described in his private diaries. For instance, in Colm Tóibín's essay on Casement's life his homosexuality is located as the crucial well-spring of Casement's sympathetic identification with the victims of imperialism and of his broadly reformist commitments. As Tóibín argued, 'perhaps it was his very homosexuality ... which made him into the humanitarian he was, made him so appalled. Unlike everyone around him he took nothing for granted. His moral courage ... came perhaps from his understanding of what it meant to be despised.'[95] At the same time, Tóibín deeply regrets the degeneration of Casement's politics from 'humanitarianism' to revolutionary activism, which to Tóibín was merely sectarian fanaticism; in his view, Casement became 'more and more anti-English as time went on and more fanatical'.

These currents persisted in the commemorative activity during 2016, from the official state commemoration held at Banna Strand in the spring through the various artistic productions during summer and autumn. As Fiona Loughnane observed, surveying various archival photographic exhibitions featuring Casement that year, 'Casement now seemed to conform to, rather than challenge, the nation's self-image'.[96] In light of the marriage referendum result the previous year, central to this conception of Casement as an icon of Irish modernity was the conception of him as a 'gay forefather'; thus, an issue of *GCN* celebrated 'Casement and the Queering of 1916'.

This belated recognition that being queer and being principally committed to anti-colonial struggle are in no way antithetical is obviously a welcome reversal of the prevailing position in Irish cultural discourse for much of the twentieth century. For decades arguments about the authenticity of Casement's diaries served as flimsy cover for a homophobic rejection of that simple proposition.[97] But is something vital also being lost here? To what degree has our recognition of Casement's sexuality come at the cost of some more challenging encounter with his revolutionary politics? Again, as so often in contemporary sexual politics, the decisive elements in this diminution of Casement's radicalism are sexual identity and its disavowed ally, sacramentalism. Nowhere in Casement's private diaries do we find him reflecting on the 'meaning' of his sexual relations, or on the significance of his erotic desires and pleasures for his self-understanding. What we find instead are coded references to men's bodies as objects of erotic desire and pleasure, and to Casement enjoying a great many sexual encounters. As we've noted, his affective and erotic responses to the bodies of men emerge in a linguistic pattern of codes (the frequent use of 'X' to indicate a sexual encounter took place), creolisation (phrases in Portuguese, Spanish, Kikongo and Irish interwoven into the predominantly English-language prose) and recurring declarative phrases: 'beautiful', 'beauties', 'beautifuls', 'beautiful types', 'lovely', 'splendid', 'enormous', 'huge', 'glorious'. In contrast with the 1903 diary, the 1910 and 1911 diaries are more explicit about Casement's sexual pleasure, and the use of 'X' is elaborated by recurring phrases: 'deep to hilt', 'enormous push', 'loved mightily', 'grand'. In short, what is of most interpretive and political interest here is not the expression of identity but a distinctive structure of feeling – encountering human bodies as sites of pleasure and vulnerability.

Nevertheless, in so much of the commemorative activity the emphasis was precisely on Casement's identity, and specifically on the hybridity of his identities. Thus, we were reminded that he was: an agent of British imperialism who became an anti-colonial insurgent; born in Dublin, but with strong familial and affective ties to Antrim; an Irish Protestant republican; a Protestant who may have become a Catholic; a nationalist who lived and worked transnationally; an Irish patriot who was queer. Some of the more facile celebration of Casement's hybridity and queerness is simply due to ill-informed and schematic views of history: ignorance of Casement's cultural nationalist milieu, for instance, in which being from a northern Protestant family and being a committed republican was not unusual; or a wholly ill-informed view of the other 1916 leaders as insular nationalists lacking any internationalist perspective – a view as ignorant of Pearse's views on bilingualism and education as of Connolly's Marxism.

But aside from those local dimensions there are also two significant ideological currents underpinning this insistence on Casement's identities over his politics. One is sacramentalism. The uneasiness, even among advocates of reclaiming Casement the 'gay forefather', with the superfluity and excess of his cruising translates into reformulating his diaries as a statement of his 'sexuality' rather than a record of erotic pleasure, and of his sexuality as having an ethical purpose through informing his understanding of oppression. Sex, in other words, must be made 'meaningful' through being ethically purposeful, and identity facilitates this. Secondly, focusing on his sexual identity produces rather blandly heroic versions of Casement that underestimate the complexity but also the actual radicalism of his political positions. In this way, he is positioned as much more amenable to the neoliberal hegemony. We can enthusiastically embrace the challenge he presents to the reactionary Catholic-nationalist formation dominant for much of the twentieth century but now largely residual, while ignoring that his reformulation as emblem of pluralism and diversity comports neatly with what is now the dominant ideology. In short, we can recuperate 'Casement' while managing to ignore the content of the historic Casement's systemic critique of global capitalism.

However, it is still striking how artists were especially drawn to remembering Casement in 2016. These artists were not always giving direct expression to Casement's anti-capitalist and anti-imperialist politics. On the contrary, their commentary on their own work generally rehearsed conventionally neoliberal and revisionist affirmations of pluralism and diversity. But fortunately, as W.H. Auden famously noted about Yeats, an artist's work is almost always much smarter than the artist themselves. Ignoring the commentary and focusing on the artwork, that work evidently tuned in to radical, insurrectionary and utopian frequencies in Casement's writing, frequencies which were simultaneously being occluded in much commemorative discourse.

Fearghus Ó Conchúir's *Butterflies and Bones* is a notable instance. In many ways, the production strove to assimilate the executed Casement to an identifiable narrative of gay injury. For instance, the male dancers' costumes evoked recognisable styles from club culture and the contemporary gay male *habitus*, thus constructing a clear identity between Casement in 1916 and a (youthful, middle-class, urban, white) gay man in 2016. Moreover, the soundscape incorporated recorded readings from official writings about, rather than by, Casement: an account of the exhumation of Casement's remains at Pentonville Prison in 1965 and an extract from the coroner's report in 1916 with graphic details of a rectal examination. The use of these texts foregrounded Casement's own body as a location of homophobic injury and martyrdom. But dance is an art form in which the human body is the medium rather than the thematic. And so, the aural affects of these spoken texts were in each case visually disrupted and challenged by the movement of the dancers' bodies on stage; by, for instance, Matthew Morris' disdainful insouciance and defiant nakedness during the reading of the 1916 extract. In this way text and performance juxtaposed different responses to the violence of capitalism: retreat to the reassurances of injury and identity, or revolt propelled by the need, vulnerability and beauty of our bodies. Distilled in that moment were different ways of remembering Casement, and different ways of reading Casement. By attending to the body being described in various states of pain and pleasure in Casement's writing, we can recognise how the revolutionary act – like the impulsive, exhilarating, speculative risk of the gambler or of the cruising man – can sometimes be the only rational response to the tragic, inhuman irrationality of capitalism.

Liberation

One of the photographs held in the Irish Queer Archive shows a group of men on O'Connell Street in Dublin.[98] Two of these men, on the viewer's right, are uniformed gardaí; one peers suspiciously at the camera while the other glances sideways. Alongside them are five men dressed in jeans and shirts or t-shirts. One man stands with his back to the camera. He is looking down O'Connell Street at the traffic and crowds in the background of the photo. Another man is smiling at the camera, posing with his hand on his hip and one leg placed slightly in front of the other, and wearing a red carnation on his patterned shirt. The photograph has a striking symmetry. The garda gazing away from the camera wears a similar moustache to the smiling man and holds his left arm at an angled position, unconsciously mirroring, in muted form, the other man's more self-consciously camp and defiant pose.

As the moustaches and the men's clothes indicate, the photograph was taken in 1984 and, more specifically, during Gay Pride Week in Dublin. The latter detail is unsurprising, since the most prominent feature in the photograph is a large banner held aloft by two of these men. It is well-crafted from a piece of pink sheer material that has been carefully cut into a triangular shape. The banner is decorated with doubled-male and doubled-female gender symbols in gold and it has the words 'Dublin Lesbian/Gay Collective' printed in large letters.

We could read this photograph as an allegory of the evolving relationship between Ireland's lesbian and gay communities and the southern Irish state in the late twentieth and early twenty-first centuries. In the photograph, the gardaí are watchfully policing the event. Their uniforms are a reminder that in 1984 sex between men was a criminal offence in the Republic of Ireland. Though that these representatives of the state appear to be tolerantly observing a Gay Pride demonstration indicates some ambivalence and inconsistency in the application of that anachronistic law. Looking at the photograph in 2021 we are reminded that in 2019 a group of uniformed gardai, alongside representatives of the Police Service of Northern Ireland (PSNI), officially participated in the Dublin Pride march. Members of the defence forces and other public services also took part, along with the then taoiseach, Leo Varadkar, and other senior politicians.

Looking again at the photograph, we notice that a sideview of the portico of the GPO features prominently. As with the circulation of Casement's iconography during the 2016 commemorations, one reading here is

that Irish lesbians and gay men have gradually assimilated into a more tolerant and pluralist Irish nation which
locates its legitimacy in the founding narrative of 1916
(of which the GPO is a visual reminder). But as we have
seen, there are other ways of thinking about, and imaginatively reconnecting with, Casement's revolutionary
politics. In the same way, we could reverse our interpretation here. Arguably, those marching gay men in the
photograph are in fact more closely aligned with the animating spirit of anticolonial revolt in 1916 – a public
act of defiance and opposition to the political and social
order – emblematised in the GPO than the two gardaí
who, conversely, emblematise the status quo. Again,
looking at the photograph in post-marriage-equality
Ireland, there are two possible interpretations of what
this image means – both requiring different imaginative
conceptions of political time from us. In the conventional historical narrative, the men stand as symbols of a
liberal modernity and of that pluralised futurity which
the Irish state has gradually embraced since 1984 – they
portend the future which we now inhabit. Alternatively,
we could argue that they symbolise a residual revolutionary current which the dominant political order strives to
supress, now just as much as in 1984; they remind us of
alternative futures that were once imaginable.

The Dublin Lesbian and Gay Collective (DLGC) was
one of several radical Irish lesbian and gay political organisations, with small overlapping memberships, active
in the first half of the 1980s. Other groupings included:

similar collectives in Cork and Galway; the Gay Defence Committee (established in response to the murder of Charles Self in 1982); Gays Against the Amendment (mobilised to support the Women's Right to Choose Campaign and oppose the constitutional amendment prohibiting abortion in 1983); and the ambitiously named Gays Against Imperialism (building alliances with left republicanism).

Recently, Maurice Casey and Patrick McDonagh – notably two historians of the younger, post-austerity generation – have recovered and re-evaluated this previously occluded moment in the history of Irish queer activism.[99] Their work is distinguished by meticulously rigorous and attentive archival scholarship, but also, and more unusually, by a dialectical political imagination which is in critical sympathy with the radical perspectives they are encountering. This is important because, as McDonagh argues, the persistent occlusion of that radical current of the Irish lesbian and gay movement – a tendency to situate it as ephemeral and marginal – in historiographical and media discourse has been politically conservative.[100] The prevailing historical narrative emphasises instead the political objective of recognition by the state (decriminalisation in 1993; marriage equality in 2015), along with the central role of non/anti-democratic institutions (such as the European Court of Human Rights) and the heroism of individuals (such as Senator David Norris) in securing that recognition. This narrative is essentially depoliticising. It discourages mobilisation – 'ordinary' people need only wait around for social change to happen – and conforms to the neo-liberal emphasis on individualised and technocratic 'solutions' to the political and economic injustice endemic to capitalist social structures.

Casey usefully outlines the factors impelling the emergence of these radical groups as alternatives to the Irish Gay Rights Movement (IGRM, founded in 1974) and the National Gay Federation (NGF, founded in 1979). The key point of dissension was the political objective of securing decriminalisation. For the NGF, securing this goal through legislative change was paramount. For the radical groups, this political effort was misapplied. As one vocal critic argued, the pursuit of decriminalisation brought attention to laws which were rarely used and must 'inevitably atrophy', while generating unfounded fear of prosecution among vulnerable members of the community.[101] More significantly, the radical groups were impatient with the exclusionary focus on decriminalisation and the narrowly defined scope of the rights being sought. From their perspective, freedom for lesbian and gay men could only be secured through a wholesale transformation of Irish society, and to achieve that it was essential to mobilise around a more expansive and radical vision of freedom while building alliances around common experiences of oppression. In other words, the divergence was one of political objectives – whether to prioritise decriminalisation – and political strategy, with the NGF focusing on media representation and lobbying while the radical groups favoured mobilising on the street. But fundamentally the divergence was ideological, and, not surprisingly, gender and class were nodal points around which those differences flared.

Two episodes in 1982 and 1983 illustrate the former. In 1982 the NGF publicly supported the Women's Right to Choose Campaign, established to resist the constitutional amendment prohibiting abortion which would be put to a referendum the following year. However, the public statement of support masked bitter internal divisions, including the argument posed by some members that taking a stance on the referendum would detract from the law reform campaign. This event exacerbated the underlying alienation of many lesbian feminist activists from the NGF's masculinist focus on gay men's rights and led to their terminal break with the organisation. On the other hand, this debate also prompted the founding of Gays Against the Amendment in response, which drew to it those gay men equally unhappy with the NGF's exclusionary politics. Likewise, the feminist commitments of the DLGC were apparent in the public demonstration protesting the lenient sentences passed on the young men responsible for Declan Flynn's murder in March 1983. Again, the demonstration indexed the difference in strategy; rather than advocating any public protest, the NGF had issued a media statement strongly condemning the verdict, but, as Casey notes, in terms 'mirroring the political mainstream's criticism'.[102] Moreover, the DLGC organisers described the protest as a march to end *sexual violence* and not only violence against gay men. Thus, the protesters marched behind a banner reading 'Stop Violence Against Women and Gays' and this point was reiterated by Cathal Kerrigan, of the DLGC, when addressing the crowd at Fairview Park.[103]

At the time, the debate about class focused on the underlying class distinctions in the lesbian and the gay movement, and especially on the predominantly middle-class, professional leadership of the NGF. The class-specific interests of the leadership, critics argued, determined the organisation's focus on recognition and a narrowly defined conception of rights.[104] But more important than the class background, and class prejudices, of individual members was the category of class relations as an analytical lens for thinking about sexual oppression under capitalism. This was a defining difference between the NGF and the DLGC, and the related radical groups. Moreover, this divergence captured at a local Irish level what has long been a central tension between two political currents in the Western lesbian and gay movement as it emerged post-Stonewall.

One strand, represented in Ireland by the DLGC and its coevals, is a universalising, liberationist and utopian political imaginary that took its coordinates from the writings of Herbert Marcuse and variants of Marxism, feminism, anti-colonialism and the New Left. From this gay liberation and lesbian feminist perspective, the struggle against the oppressive stigmatisation of homosexuality is necessarily inseparable from the struggle for a revolution in which all social institutions – notably private property, marriage and the family – and all social relations – gender, race, class – would be radically transformed. In this view, sexuality was not an autonomous category of 'private' experience but embedded in the matrix of capitalist social relations. This was a revolutionary objective which aimed to undermine wholesale the modern sex-gender system. Liberation required the radical transformation not just of social structures and norms but, just as essentially, those forms of consciousness, with their supporting ideological binaries, within which homosexuality functioned as the antonym of heterosexuality. If liberation was aimed at ending patriarchy, and therefore heterosexuality, as a category of identity, then it would of necessity bring about 'the end of the homosexual', as Dennis Altman predicted in his pioneering manifesto of the 'gay lib' position.[105] 'Gay liberation' was less about the freedom to be gay than the freedom to be neither gay nor straight.

The other strand in the post-Stonewall movement is a reformist or assimilative liberal/social democratic project seeking recognition, protection and civil rights for a lesbian and gay minority. This is predicated on a formative connection between erotic desire and identity, the notion that each of us 'has' a 'sexuality', as well as the relative autonomy of sexuality from other social relations. It assumes the continued existence of a fundamental hetero–homo binary, albeit one more tolerantly mediated by cultural norms and, where that fails, actively policed by the state to ensure parity. In short, freedom from oppression for lesbians and gay men can, in this view, be secured within the existing social order; indeed, it can only really be secured within the dominant liberal democratic and capitalist order.

We can gain some fascinating insight into this tension between minoritarianism/reformism and universalism/radicalism in the Irish lesbian and gay movement from a leading activist whose commitments straddled these perspectives, and who wrote as an organic intellectual striving for a coherent synthesis of them. Kieran Rose's *Diverse Communities: The evolution of lesbian and gay politics in Ireland* was published in 1994, a year after decriminalisation was achieved in the republic. Rose provides a precisely detailed but lively account of the lobbying campaign in the late 1980s and early 1990s directed towards securing decriminalisation. This account is intimately informed by his prominent role in that campaign. At the same time, he is keen to situate the achievement of decriminalisation as just one, albeit significant, strand in the concerns, objectives and achievements of the Irish lesbian and gay movement. His perspective in the book has a double orientation: towards the past, to understand the gradual formation of a political consciousness and mobilisation of energies leading to 1993; towards the future, identifying pressing needs and political goals demanding continuing effort.

Rose argues that the Irish lesbian and gay movement evolved distinctively. It took its coordinates from metropolitan developments and models while at the same time articulating with radical anti-imperialist and socialist republican traditions within Irish history. For Rose, decriminalisation was a belated act of decolonisation. The laws annulled in 1993, dating from 1861 and 1885, had been passed in the Westminster parliament and retained on the statute books after 1922. As Rose reiterates, the retention of the laws was symptomatic of the counter-revolutionary tenor dominant in the two new states on the partitioned island. More speculatively, Rose argues that institutionalised homophobia was a colonial implant in Ireland and other colonies, alluding to the Brehon Laws and other evidence that Gaelic Ireland was more tolerant of same-sex relationships.

Rose believes that during the twenty years before decriminalisation people began to 'construct a new identity which meant that it is possible to be Irish *and* lesbian *and* gay'.[106] He is keen to challenge the notion that decriminalisation was enforced or imposed on the country by Europe, which he argues was a narrative peddled by right-wing activists. While the finding of the European Court of Human Rights in 1988, in favour of David Norris' case against the constitutionality of the law, compelled the Irish state to act, Rose is keen to stress that the 1993 law reform was far more extensive, progressive and egalitarian than the similar law reform in Britain in 1967. This outcome, he demonstrates, had less to do with the court judgement than with fertile conditions in Irish politics. These included strategic opportunities for alliance-building (the support of trade unions and the Irish Council for Civil Liberties), support from key institutions, such as the Law Reform Commission, and key figures in political parties. Above all, Rose claims, this egalitarian and progressive reform was possible because of 'positive traditional Irish values arising from the anti-colonial struggle reinvigorated and amplified by the new social, cultural and economic influences of the 1960s onwards'.[107]

Rose's analysis of the oppression of lesbian and gay people is manifestly informed by socialist and anti-capitalist commitments, foregrounding the necessity of transforming society structurally to achieve sexual liberation for all. Thus, for instance, his historical account of Irish gay and lesbian activism in the 1970s and 1980s particularly highlights the role of the smaller radical organisations, especially the Cork and Dublin gay and lesbian collectives of which he was a member. But at the same time, his account is primarily taken up with describing the political activities of the Gay and Lesbian Equality Network (GLEN). As Rose puts it, GLEN 'evolved' from the movement of the 1970s and 1980s and in 1988 was 'given the remit to campaign for equality'.[108] As the vagueness of this passive locution suggests – who exactly did the 'giving'? – the *modus operandi* was no longer collective mobilisation but a small, highly focused group speaking *for* a minority and mediating between that minority and the wider society. The chosen political terrain would now be the nexus of media, academia, non-governmental organisations, state bodies and party politics where policy is formulated, public opinion nudged in required directions and politicians and civil servants lobbied through multiple forums of varying transparency. The central objective was not revolutionary transformation of the social order but the attainment of 'equality' within the existing social and economic structures.

However, missing from Rose's account is any sense of the larger political context in which the ascendency of gay and lesbian assimilationism took place. When GLEN was remaking the Irish lesbian and gay movement along reformist lines from 1988, it was also adapting to what was then becoming the chief political mode of contemporary Irish politics. The pluralist and consensual politics exemplified by the achievement of decriminalisation, and the subsequent creation of the Equality Authority in 1999, was also the ideological basis for what was known as social partnership which took shape at almost exactly the same time as GLEN's emergence. The Programme for National Recovery was agreed between the government, the trade unions and employer organisations in 1987. This was the first of six triannual agreements through which Irish governments gained consent from the sectoral groups for government policy on public spending, pay and labour relations. During the 1990s and 2000s social partnership was ritually celebrated by mainstream economists and centrist political commentators for providing the 'stability' deemed essential for economic prosperity. However, analysis from Marxist, world-systems theory and other critical perspectives convincingly debunked this myth. For one thing, rather than social partnership generating economic growth, its primary function was to create the conditions – low taxation; low public spending; pliant, 'flexible' labour force – for the integration of Ireland into a globalising world economy. In other words, the achievement was not a dynamic economy – as its cheerleaders claimed – but a dependent economy, in which democratic control was thoroughly subordinated to the priorities and demands of global capital. Moreover, under the comforting illusion of consensus the corporatist structures of social partnership undermined representative democracy since control over significant elements of social policy shifted from the political realm into more opaque bureaucratic processes. Social partnership, as Peadar Kirby argued in 2001, 'marks an emasculation of politics as power is more concentrated in the hands of small elites and it is these who decide who gets a seat at the decision-making table'.[109] Crucially, through controlling wages in an era of accelerated expansion of profits, the agreements effectively facilitated the redistribution of wealth, on a very significant scale, from the majority of Irish citizens to local and global elites.[110]

There are two points of note here. One is the degree to which social partnership exemplified the central characteristics of neoliberal governance. Recasting the Irish state as a neoliberal rather than a democratic state – that is, a state whose primary goal is to sustain and protect the market rather than any democratic notion of the public good – was never a political objective for which politicians campaigned or citizens voted, and nor was it forced on those citizens. Instead, the majority consented – literarily, in the case of workers, through their trade unions – to this diminution of their rights as citizens because such consent *felt* like either a positive affirmation (moving beyond outmoded class antagonism to 'partnership' and 'solidarity') or an unavoidable submission to 'common sense' – or some combination of these. Moreover, the cultural discourses constructing this 'common sense' signified political dynamics in individualised and moralised terms; thus, demanding higher pay was cast as 'selfishness'. Secondly, the affinity between the institutional apparatus and discourses of social partnership and the mode of minoritarian politics pursued by GLEN points to a significant contradiction: the mainstream of lesbian and gay politics was successfully pursuing the goal of equality within Irish society just as inequality was being systematically re-entrenched in that society. Was this merely coincidence? Or was the concept of equality subtending lesbian and gay politics actually compatible with – useful for the purposes of – the ideology producing inequality?

As Maurice Casey argues, there were also other factors determining the decline of radical lesbian and gay political organising in Ireland from the mid-1980s.[111] One was the economic recession and the consequent flow of emigrants, especially the younger generation, from the country. Another was a generalised demoralisation among liberals, progressives and radicals – and, most acutely, feminists – precipitated by defeat for the progressive campaigns in two referendums (1983 and 1986, the latter on lifting the ban on divorce). The referendum defeats were symptoms of a more pervasive right-wing reaction against the feminist and liberalising achievements of the 1970s. This counter-reaction was led by the Catholic Church and right-wing lay Catholics in Ireland but was also a local manifestation of a secular trend across the (especially Anglophone) West. Most acutely for lesbian and gay radical activists, the emergence of the AIDS catastrophe, as a generation of gay men began to fall ill and die, shifted their political focus towards more immediate needs and the struggle to create an infrastructure of support services in an inhospitable, homophobic environment. In a world so cruelly foreshortened for many gay men it became difficult to imagine any future let alone a radically transformed one. More specifically, Irish state agencies cited the 1885 laws as a legal obstacle to working with the community to actively develop support structures and AIDS prevention measures. And so, for urgent reasons, the radical activists were forced to re-evaluate their position on the political priority of decriminalisation.

Two points are worth noting here. Firstly, the activist response to the AIDS crisis is a compelling demonstration of how the human body as a location of need and vulnerability, rather than a psychological and social conception of identity, can provide a powerful impetus to political mobilisation. Secondly, my characterisation of some absolute distinction between a minoritarian, assimilationist and reformist lesbian and gay politics, on one side, and a universalist, radical and revolutionary sexual politics on the other is a misleading simplification. As Kieran Rose's narrative demonstrates, while the denominated radical groups ceased to exist in the mid-1980s, their members did not always or necessarily abandon politics but recommitted themselves to other objectives. The groups disappeared but the political vision inspiring them did not, and revolutionary energies fuelled the pursuit of reformist ends. Again, looking closer to our own time, as we saw in the 'Vulnerability' section above, Una Mullally's account of the campaign for marriage equality demonstrates how precisely this dynamic was operative in the new millennium. But if securing marriage rights was, as many of its advocates argue, the capstone to the forty-year pursuit of those minoritarian and reformist objectives, this might present a welcome opportunity. Untrammelled by the necessity of achieving immediate relief from discrimination, perhaps those revolutionary energies could now be re-harnessed to a more expansive, transformative and liberationist political ambition?

As I have been speculating in this essay, that realignment in sexual politics towards universalist and revolutionary demands requires an ethical and political reorientation: from desires to needs; from identities to bodies; from injuries to vulnerabilities. Or, to draw on

Marcuse's formulation in *Eros and Civilisation* (1955), from sexuality to Eros. As Marcuse argued, in capitalist society, what we term sexuality is the human capacity for pleasure and intimacy subordinated to the performance principle. 'Sexuality', in Marcuse's conception of the term, describes a human instinct narrowly inhibited and confined to genital activity and reproduction, and restricted to a socially and morally sanctified realm of marriage and the patriarchal family. This conceptualisation of sexuality has been inseparable from those rigid binaries underpinning bourgeois subjectivity: between the body as productive instrument and the creative soul or mind; between labour and leisure; between a masculine public sphere and a feminine private sphere; between political and moral actions; between individual relations and social relations. In other words, sexuality, in Marcuse's usage, is inseparable from the reification of human consciousness, affects and relationships under capitalism. The 'organisation of sexuality' – the centralisation of the libidinal instincts into one object of desire, embodied in a member of the opposite sex, which defines the formation of healthy, 'normal' subjectivity in the Freudian narrative – requires the 'desexualisation of the body: the libido becomes concentrated in one part of the body, leaving most of the rest free for use as instrument of labour'.[112]

Central to Marcuse's utopian vision of a 'non-repressive civilisation' – a human culture freed from the domination of the performance principle – that we might strive to imagine and create, is the distinction he draws between 'sexuality' and 'Eros'. In a non-repressive culture, Eros would describe a state where the human body 'no longer used as a full-time instrument of labour would be resexualised ... the body in its entirety would be an object of cathexis, a thing to be enjoyed – an instrument of pleasure'. For Marcuse, the transformation of sexuality into Eros should not be thought of simply in terms of individual psyches throwing off the shackles of repressive morality, 'sexual liberation' as the 1960s counterculture understood it, but of a revolutionary reordering of social relations. This will require, he reiterates, 'not simply a release but a transformation of libido; from sexuality constrained under genital supremacy to eroticisation of the entire personality'. This transformation of human consciousness will be the result of 'a societal transformation that released the play of individual needs and faculties'.[113]

Returning to the thought of one of gay liberation's inspirational forefathers reminds us that a radical political realignment requires not only a transformation in the lexicon of our political demands but also a complex temporal reorientation. We must learn to refuse the regimented linearity of liberal progress and capitalist modernisation. Instead, we must cultivate a hopeful longing for a transformed future while simultaneously journeying into the past to find nourishing sustenance for our political imagination – encountering ghostly reminders, in places like the DLGC archives, that other futures were once possible and may still be.

Hope

In April and May 2015 one image developed a very significant media currency – in Ireland and internationally – as an expressive signifier of the marriage equality campaign. Joe Caslin's 'The Claddagh Embrace' was an image of two men embracing, which Caslin created as a large-scale mural on the gable wall of a five-storey building in Dublin city centre, at the busy junction of South Great George's Street and Dame Street, and thus opposite the city's longest-established gay bar (see Figure 1). Caslin also created a fourteen-metre-high mural on the wall of Caher Castle, the remains of a late-medieval tower house in rural County Galway; there the image was of two women embracing. Together the images formed Caslin's intervention in support of a 'yes' vote in the referendum. In 2016 he also created a large-scale mural, portraying two women kissing, on a wall in Belfast to draw attention to the ongoing campaign for marriage equality in Northern Ireland.[114]

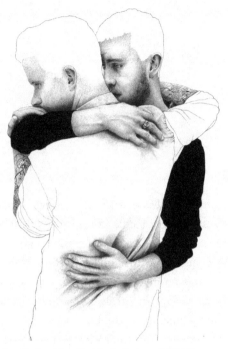

Figure 1: Joe Caslin, 'The Claddagh Embrace' (2015)

Caslin describes his artistic practice as explicitly political and activist. In 'Our Nation's Sons', for instance, he created a series of portraits of working-class boys and young men in various urban locations around Ireland and in Edinburgh. The project, created over five years, addressed the media stereotyping of these young men and the prevalence of mental health disorders, self-harm and suicide among them. In 2016 one of his largest murals – on a seven-storey vacant hotel overlooking Waterford city – also addressed the prevalence of male

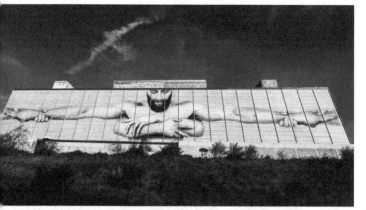

Figure 2: Joe Caslin, 'Ar Scáth a Chéile a Mhaireann na Daoine' ('We Live Protected Under Each Other's Shadow') (2016). Photo by Peter Grogan/Emagine.

suicide. 'Ar Scáth a Chéile a Mhaireann na Daoine' ('We Live Protected Under Each Other's Shadow') shows a bearded male figure with downcast eyes and outstretched arms; each of his hands is clasped by the hands of unseen figures whose arms stretch from the margins of the mural. The central figure is also being embraced from behind, and again we only see the arms of this embracing figure clasped tightly across the man's naked torso (see Figure 2).

Likewise, Caslin has collaborated on 'The Volunteers', a multi-media project 'highlighting the importance of volunteerism in tackling some of Ireland's most pressing issues: drug addiction, mental health, and direct provision'.[115] In the first part of the project Caslin created a mural on a building at Trinity College, in 2017, specifically addressing the criminalisation of drug use, and the attendant diversion of resources from care and treatment. There are four figures: three women (Rachael Keogh and Fiona O'Reilly, who work in the field, and Senator Lynn Ruane, who introduced legislation to decriminalise drug use) and a male figure representing a doctor turning away from the women. One of the women is dressed as a nurse, but the style of her uniform is reminiscent of the early twentieth century. Likewise, the doctor's formal clothes (hat, overcoat, wing-collar and tie) are vaguely Edwardian. The historical allusions play on the references to 1916 in the project title. This idea, contemporary political activists as heirs to the spirit of the Easter Rising, is foregrounded more directly in the short video on which Caslin collaborated. Over a montage (Caslin working on his drawing; the mural being erected; drug use; inner city neighbourhoods; Glasnevin cemetery) an actress, Ally Ni Chiarain, recites a poem – 'We Will Let No Life Be Worth Less' – written for the project by Erin Fornoff: 'The new volunteers/a nation reflected/its warrior creed: "We will be fierce in our compassion and believe"'.[116]

A second mural in 'The Volunteers' project was erected on the wall of the National Museum of Ireland at Collins Barracks in Dublin. It shows two young men, facing each other in a crouched position. One looks out at the viewer, while holding the other man; the latter's gaze is towards the ground as he leans his head against the other's chest and supports his arms on the other's shoulders (see Figure 3). Caslin identified the men as '20-year-old

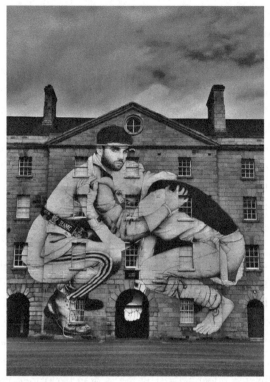

Figure 3: Joe Caslin, 'The Volunteers – Collins Barracks' (2017)

GAA athlete and volunteer Cormac Coffey and Eanna Walsh, a 28-year-old man who in 2014 was diagnosed with bipolar disorder'.[117] One assumes that Cormac is the figure gazing outward, his unflinching gaze indexing the physical and emotional strength which he can impart to the suffering Eanna. However, the awkward physical position in which they are posed means that the two men are literally supporting each other to stay upright; in other words, the pose suggests interdependence rather than any unidirectional, and paternalistic, transfer of support from 'carer' to 'client'.

Caslin's posing of the lovers in 'The Claddagh Embrace', along with their anxious mood, explicitly referenced Frederic William Burton's 'Hellelil and Hildebrand, the Meeting on the Turret Stairs' (1864), a Pre-Raphaelite-style watercolour depicting a scene from a medieval Danish ballad. In a 'poll' conducted by the National Gallery of Ireland in 2012, this painting was 'voted' as 'the nation's favourite' and this popularity was one reason why Caslin chose to allude to it.[118] In 2017–18 Caslin had a residency at the National Gallery, in conjunction with an exhibition of Burton's work, and the result of this was a project entitled 'Finding Power'. This included a sequence of seven photographic portraits. Those portrayed included: a politician, a comedian, two people who had come to Ireland as an asylum seeker and a refugee respectively; an academic and disability rights activist; a queer activist/writer; a drag performer. Each portrait incorporates a plinth and various gold-coloured accessories or objects, and the stylised poses echo motifs and conventions of classical statuary and post-Renaissance portraiture. Caslin reproduced one of these photographs, of Stephen Moloney, as a highly finished graphite and ink drawing, which was then installed as a large-scale mural in the gallery.[119]

Taken together, Caslin's work has manifest critical and progressive political commitments and these are expressed through his choice of subjects, his collaborations and his framing of the work in media interviews and public talks. At the same time, there is an even more radical political perspective latently embedded in the form and style of his images. This radical potential takes shape through the recurring dialectic of power and vulnerability. Caslin's monochrome line drawings are delicate, refined and sparse, and yet the murals confront the viewer forcefully because of their size. Intimate images of the human form are projected on a startlingly inhuman scale. The murals are aesthetically disconcerting. The realist style – reminiscent of early Soviet-era social realism, with its 'ordinary' figures posed heroically – is undermined by the expressionism of contorted bodies and enigmatic gazes. The realism is further distorted by the scale and puzzling hybridity of the form (neither fresco nor poster nor digital projection but adapting some texture from each).

This discombobulating affect is reiterated through the position of the murals. The viewer does not go looking for these art works in spaces that are designated for contemplating art. Instead, the murals find their viewers, and surprise them, as they go about their daily lives; like Walter Benjamin's revolutionary memory flashing up at a moment of danger, Caslin's murals rise up unexpectedly from the cityscape and landscape.[120] In this way the content of the images portray the human form as vulnerable, while their form – monumental scale; hybrid styles; unexpected appearance – makes the viewer viscerally conscious of their own vulnerability. Moreover, by wresting a space of aesthetic experience and political contemplation from the dominated space of capitalism, Caslin engages in the potentially revolutionary act of appropriating space by resituating the human body in a dynamic and relational encounter with the space it creates.

This distinction between dominated and appropriated space was drawn by Henri Lefebvre in his pioneering elaboration of the concept of social space. For Lefebvre, the purpose of thinking about how we apprehend space is to uncover the social relationships embedded in it. The social relations of production, he argued, have a social existence to the extent that they have a spatial existence. Dominated space describes a space that is transformed, and mediated, by technology; dominated space, as Lefebvre observes, is 'closed, sterilised, emptied out'.[121] By contrast, appropriated space is 'modified in order to serve the needs and possibilities of a group' and so 'appropriative activity is creative rather than dominating'. The history of capitalist development, according to Lefebvre, has been a history of mutual antagonism between these forms of occupying space and 'the winner in this context has been domination'.[122]

Caslin's portraits of the male body – a significant motif in his work – engage directly with those cultural ideals framing hegemonic masculinity as aggressively competitive and autonomous, and with the damage these discourses inflict on young men specifically. Thus, for instance, the images comprising 'Our Nation's Sons' repeatedly show the young men wearing a hooded sweatshirt or hoodie. Their clothing acts as a signifier of their stigmatised lack of respectability and of how they, and those of their class, are perceived as dangerous – the view that hoodies provide anonymising disguise for criminality. Yet the posture of the young men shows them wearing those hoodies less as armour, an assertive gesture of aggression, than as a protective shield; a co-cooning, womblike space in which to hide. In 'Ar Scáth a Chéile a Mhaireann na Daoine' ('We Live Protected Under Each Other's Shadow') and the 'Finding Power' image of Stephen Moloney magnified for the National Gallery installation, this vulnerability is conveyed through the contorted posing of the body: disproportionate out-stretched arms; awkwardly arranged limbs; twisted torso. But that vulnerability merges with a mood of resilience and powerfulness that is not conveyed as assertive-ness but as easeful contemplation (closed eyes; averted gaze). Above all, that vulnerability of the male body is registered as relationality and dependence. Thus, for instance, in the Waterford mural the image of the restful body supported by the arms of the other literalises Judith Butler's observation that 'the body is not, and never was, a self-subsisting kind of being ... the body is given over to others in order to persist; it is given over to some other set of hands before it can make use of its own'.[123]

Strikingly, these images depict the beauty and erotic energy of the male body, but not a male body armoured in musculature. Caslin's images affectingly counter that signifier of male desirability through which the performance principle is erotically embodied: sculpted bodies as the exchange value extracted from the relentless labour to 'produce' such results. As we saw with Paul Ryan's interlocuters, while such images of the male body have high, and monetised, value in contemporary gay male culture, they are in fact circulating everywhere in contemporary visual culture. Moreover, the vulnerability inhering in Caslin's images of the male body reminds us how the expectation that one should inhabit an aggressively competitive autonomy is not just specific to masculine identity. Rather it is woven into the hegemonic conception of subjectivity as such, the ideal of the entrepreneurial self, valorised in neoliberal culture.[124]

More than just signifiers of an alternative masculine identity, Caslin's male bodies are what Ernst Bloch termed 'guiding images' of a radical humanism – gesturing towards the radical potential of vulnerability and dependence to reorientate our political imaginary. For Bloch, a guiding image is a cultural figure or type imaginatively embodying an idealised form of human subjectivity to which we might aspire – an imaginative realisation of our potentialities. For him, the most powerful guiding image of modernity is the *citoyen* first imagined by Marx, a figure that 'rose up in contrast to the egotistical individual member of bourgeois society'. By contrast with the ideal of bourgeois individualism, the *citoyen* 'was conceived as a member of a non-egotistical and therefore still imaginary *polis*. He was idealised as the other side of the bourgeois, and thus, in his non-egotistical dreamlike beauty, not subject to the division of labour and not reified, he was idealised with particular force'.[125]

In creating his murals Caslin affixes the drawings to the building using biodegradable materials. This intentional transience weaves vulnerability, such a key symbolic element in his imagery, into the material fabric of the work. This material transience of the artwork encodes a revolutionary perspective on history – a sense of time as open, and of present and future as dynamic and plastic. Likewise, that open historical perspective is reiterated through Caslin's incorporation of allusions to political and art history, and, most notably, his incorporation of structures of feeling that take their coordinates from religious iconography (the Waterford mural alluding to art-historical crucifixion scenes, for instance) and anti-colonial nationalism. This is daring, since in the liberal and progressive Irish political discourse that embraces Caslin, and from which he takes his coordinates, those 'traditional' structures of feeling are conventionally held to be irredeemably discredited by their association with conservative and oppressive institutions.

Again, Bloch's circuitously expansive philosophical mediations on political hope, his demonstration that the cultivation of hope is indispensable for the utopian imaginary, is a useful frame for thinking about these curious temporal dimensions of Caslin's work. Bloch reiterates that hope is always both cognitive and emotional, or more precisely affective; it merges the 'cold stream' of analysis with the 'warm stream' of imagination, thereby requiring us to challenge the ideological binary of cognition and affect. Moreover, the cultivation of hope requires the cultivation of an alternative standpoint on reality than that promulgated by the rationality of capitalist realism. To be (politically) hopeful is to be alert not just to what is, but also to the 'not-yet-become' – those 'anticipatory elements which are a component of reality itself' – and to the 'not-yet-conscious', which, for Bloch, is the creative capacity that allows us to anticipate the 'not-yet-become' as an open possibility.[126] This requires a conception of the world as 'unenclosed', and therefore of reality as 'process', and of 'the widely ramified mediation between present, unfinished past and, above all, possible future'.[127]

Like Bloch, Marcuse also stresses the indispensable role of imagination and fantasy when striving to fulfil the potential to create revolutionised forms of consciousness and social relations. Art provides imaginative projections of a freedom that can only yet exist in potential, not realised, form; it expresses 'the return of the repressed image of liberation'.[128] Reflecting on Caslin's images of the male form, it is notable that Marcuse pays particular attention to artistic images and narratives of the male body as figures for envisioning the potential of Eros and of a non-repressive culture. Specifically, Marcuse examines the representation of three mythological figures – Christ, Orpheus and Narcissus – in which the male body has been depicted as simultaneously vulnerable and beautiful; as we have seen, the history of artistic images of Christ and Narcissus (the latter most notably in the National Gallery of Ireland portrait of Stephen Moloney) are important intertextual allusions in Caslin's work.

In Marcuse's interpretation, Christ articulated a 'message of liberation: the overthrow of the Law (which is domination) by Agape (which is Eros)'.[129] The most powerful symbol of this message was Christ becoming human and bodily, and making himself vulnerable to suffering – hence the recurrence of crucifixion imagery in Western art. According to Marcuse, Christ's followers subsequently betrayed that message of liberation by constructing a narrative emphasising Christ's transubstantiation and deification, what Marcuse terms 'the denial of the liberation in the flesh'.[130] This orthodox Christian version of Christ as transcending the limitations of the body became one of Western civilisation's most powerful symbolic vehicles for that damaging hierarchy of body subordinated to mind/soul, which took secular form in the reification of consciousness under capitalism. For Marcuse, the revision of the Greek myth of Narcissus in psychoanalysis further reaffirmed that same binary of body and mind/soul by translating an image of sensuous male beauty into a moral tale of fatal, self-destructive vanity. This moralism was given 'scientific' validation in the adaptation of the myth into Freudian and neo-Freudian 'explanations' of homosexuality, and such ideas still circulate in popular stereotypes of gay men. Again, Marcuse revises the tale, noting that Narcissus did not know that the image he admired was his own. Thus, rather than an image of the self-absorbed separative self, Narcissus' pleasurable contemplation of his own beauty depicts a relational standpoint, an openness to the other and to the natural world he inhabits. Marcuse observes the 'striking paradox that narcissism, usually understood as egotistical withdrawal from reality, is here connected with oneness with the universe ... narcissism denotes a fundamental relatedness to reality which may generate a comprehensive existential order'.[131]

Marcuse's distinction between sexuality and Eros can also be formulated temporally. In the Freudian narrative of self-development which Marcuse was challenging, for each of us to become a functioning human subject polymorphous perversity must be left behind and our perverse desires must be brought under control and diverted into genital procreative – (re)productive – sexuality. In this view, the formation of the self is stadial (the ego passing through various stages of development, most notably the Oedipal complex) and teleological – there is a definite endpoint, which is a 'normal' self in conformity with the repressive demands of civilisation. In this, the Freudian narrative is strikingly similar to the developmental historicism underpinning imperialism and capitalism; societies must also pass through stages of primitivism and 'underdevelopment' to become functioning capitalist economies. For Marcuse, by contrast, the temporality of perversity is prophetic rather than progressive. The wilfulness and excess of eroticism is not what needs to be left behind, but that which offers a suggestive glimpse of future possibilities – an image of what Eros, liberation, might be like. Like fantasy, to which it is closely aligned, perversity is a 'revolt against the performance principle in the name of the pleasure principle' and thus a residue of the pre-social consciousness offering a glimpse of what sexuality transformed into Eros might look like in the future.[132] And, reflecting on the similarities between Freud's normative model of the self and imperialist ideology, we might recall the political undercurrents of cruising in Casement's writing and its symbolic alignment with the recalcitrant temporality of anti-colonial revolt.

Reflecting on Caslin's 'The Claddagh Embrace' – on the tenderness and vulnerability of the image, and then the history of its political potency in the marriage referendum – confronts us with the dilemma of thinking politically about that paradoxical conjunction – 'marriage equality' – and its contradictions: the achievement of equality within a rigidly unequal political and economic order. As we observed, that contradiction was given affective expression in that very different image of intimacy between men, the 'Viva School of Dance' ad, with which we began. One possible response to this contradiction is to redouble our commitment to the politics of identity, diversity and recognition.

For instance, this is the position adopted by Emer O'Toole in her critique of the 'yes' campaign. O'Toole offers a perceptive account of the evolving discussion of 'gay marriage' in Irish media discourse in the years leading up to 2015. Paradigmatic here was the media persona of the drag-activist Panti Bliss. That persona, O'Toole argues, could be simultaneously transgressive and persuasively reassuring for an Irish audience. O'Toole underscores how the framing of homophobia in Irish media discourse illustrates that the ideological lacunae of liberalism can provide succour for conservatives, in this case a group of conservative activists very handsomely compensated, out of public money, for the 'injury' of being named as homophobic.[133] Her central criticism of the 'yes' campaign is that it did not counter the pervasive imagery of heterosexual families circulated by the 'No' campaign, and so it secured its victory through complicity with the homophobia prevalent in the society.

One major difficulty with O'Toole's analysis is that the politics of recognition displaces any attention to the functioning of ideology. The neoliberal politics of marriage rights becomes reducible to the liberal politics of representation. Thus, the 'yes' campaigners are culpable because they 'disguised queer subjectivities and queer kinship, and by extension they disguised queer politics'.[134] The emphasis is on visibility and marginalisation. As is so often the case in a certain post-deconstructionist style of queer theory, the category of 'queer' is contradictory. It is simultaneously represented as a radical standpoint on identity as such and as constituting in itself another category of identity. In an ironic twist, queer, once a tool for deconstructing what Butler in *Gender Trouble* famously termed the 'metaphysics of substance', culturally ingrained conceptions of a human essence, has somehow become a guarantor of authenticity: those categorising themselves as 'queer' being more authentic than those who, being 'merely' lesbian or gay, find themselves hopelessly inauthenticated by their unthinking aspiration to 'homonormativity'.[135] Strikingly, this vanguardism co-exists in O'Toole's analysis with a strategic temporal lag. In a telling aside, she notes that after a few days 'The Claddagh Embrace' bore traces of an egg which was thrown at it. For O'Toole, this is yet another instance of the censorship which Panti Bliss was subjected to on RTÉ. In an Irish context formulating a political question in terms of censorship, and resistance to it, is to implicitly evoke the mid-twentieth-century decades when censorship legislation was very actively and oppressively used by the post-independence state to supress intellectual life and, in particular, to supress discussion of sexuality. The implication is that nothing really has changed. This may be demoralising – or it may be remarkably reassuring. If our political positions can be formulated in familiar terms of oppressive institutions and oppressed or marginalised minorities, we are spared the difficult, challenging work of thinking dialectically about the actual hegemonic norms shaping our lives, political perspectives and identities.

The narrative arc of O'Toole's analysis elides the very significant gap in cultural capital between the person who threw the egg – by any standards a hostile but impotent gesture – and those with control over, and access to, cultural and political institutions such as the national broadcaster, RTÉ. Thus, politics is framed in statically minoritarian terms – an homogenously oppressive majority of 'them' aligned against an equally homogenised minority of the queer 'us' – in which the dynamic structure of class relations, and the neoliberal ideology underpinning contemporary capitalism, disappear from view. We might note two ironies here. One is that Panti Bliss (and O'Neill) is, in this view, an exemplary figure of the marginalised queer minority and yet, as O'Toole's discussion illustrates, has considerable access to institutions such as RTÉ and the Abbey Theatre; in short, he has access to considerably greater cultural capital and power than the anonymous egg thrower, who is nevertheless, in O'Toole's schema, exemplary of that powerful majority. The second irony is that the anonymous egg thrower was, in all probability, somebody very like the alienated boys and young men whose lives Caslin so sympathetically evoked in 'Our Nation's Sons'. The point, of course, is not to reverse the polarities – Panti Bliss is 'really' powerful; the anonymous egg thrower is 'really' marginalised – but to note how this minor instance illustrates more generally the futility of this calculus of *ressentiment* to which minoritarian identity politics can lead.

To put this another way, there are different ways of 'looking' at 'The Claddagh Embrace', and these ways of looking illustrate contrasting possibilities for a future politics of sexuality in late capitalist Ireland. O'Toole focuses on the hostility directed towards Caslin's mural and thereby frames this image of two men embracing as expressive of, as defined by, injury. As essayed above, my way of looking has been to frame Caslin's murals in terms of vulnerability, where, as we discussed earlier, vulnerability is an affective and aesthetic mode that also encodes a radical and hopeful political imaginary.

The divergence between those ways of looking can also stand for the defining choice confronting sexual politics in contemporary Ireland. One option is to persist with the form of politics which culminated in the securing of marriage rights for same-sex relationships, along with the various other forms of recognition and protection secured since 1993, while making that politics just a bit more 'queer' and diverse by reformulating the vocabulary but not the political grammar of the demand for recognition. The alternative is to grasp those achievements since 1993 (or 1974, actually) dialectically – neither the ultimate apotheosis of 'equality' nor a betrayal to the forces of homophobia, but a paradoxical victory that simultaneously made the society more equal and more unequal. Just such a dialectical perspective on the past can inform a radically hopeful perspective on the future.

Crucially it can help us to see our way to a different form of politics: a politics universal and radically humanist in its imaginative scope, and anti-capitalist and revolutionary in its objectives. Art like Joe Caslin's murals does not provide solutions to that dilemma, nor roadmaps for the political future – nor should we require it to do so. What art can provide are guiding images prompting us towards imagining less alienated, more humane and sustainable ways of being human – imagining 'a mode of being that has absorbed all becoming, that is for and with itself in all otherness'.[136]

Notes and References

(All URLs are valid at time of going to press)

1. Páraic Kerrigan and Maria Pramaggiore, 'Homoheroic or Homophobic? Leo Varadkar, LGBTQ politics and contemporary news narratives', *Critical Studies in Media Communication*, vol. 38, no. 2, 2021, pp. 107–26.

2. Kerrigan and Pramaggiore describe homoheroism as a recent phenomenon within political and popular culture. It 'refers to the expression of a range of affirming attitudes towards LGBTQ public figures' and, more specifically, 'celebrates the bravery of being an out public figure' (p. 111). Political figures in this category include: Jóhanna Sigurðardóttir, prime minister of Iceland from 2009 to 2013; Xavier Bettel, elected prime minister of Luxembourg in 2013; Ana Brnabić, appointed Serbian prime minister in 2017; and Pete Buttigieg, who contested the Democratic primaries during the US presidential election campaign in 2020 and was subsequently appointed to the US cabinet under the Biden administration.

3. David Alderson, *Sex, Needs and Queer Culture: From liberation to the post-*gay (London: Zed Books, 2016), pp. 83–93.

4. Anna MacCarthy and Aoife O'Driscoll, 'Leo Varadkar Will Be as Helpful to the Gays as Margaret Thatcher Was to Women', *GCN*, 6 June 2017, https://gcn.ie/leo-varadkar-margaret-thatcher. See also Una Mullally, 'Varadkar Election a Strange One for LGBT People', *Irish Times*, 5 June 2017, https://www.irishtimes.com/opinion/varadkar-election-a-strange-one-for-lgbt-people-1.3107615. For an excellent overview of these responses to Varadkar's election, see Brian Finnegan, 'The Varadkar Paradox', *GCN*, no. 332, August 2017, https://pocketmags.com/eu/gcn-magazine/332/articles/179754/the-varadkar-paradox. *GCN* (formerly *Gay Community News*) is a Dublin-based not-for-profit publication which has been published by a voluntary organisation, the National Lesbian and Gay Federation (NXF), continuously since 1988.

5. Wendy Brown, 'American Nightmare: Neoliberalism, neoconservatism, and de-democratisation', *Political Theory*, vol. 34, no. 6, 2006, p. 698.

6. Sarah Bardon, 'Varadkar Wants to Lead Party for "People Who Get Up Early in the Morning"', *Irish Times*, 20 May 2017, https://www.irishtimes.com/news/politics/varadkar-wants-to-lead-party-for-people-who-get-up-early-in-the-morning-1.3090753.

7. Brown, 'American Nightmare', pp. 703–5.

8. It is worth noting that MacCarthy and O'Driscoll raise this point in their article.

9. This style of radical temporal reasoning – what she terms 'periods of potent possibility' and 'avant-garde nostalgia' – is also explored by Heather Laird in *Commemoration* (Cork: Cork University Press, 2018), pp. 30–8, 58–66.

10. Two Fuse, *Freedom?* (Cork: Cork University Press, 2018), p. 55.

11. Tom Inglis, *Moral Monopoly: The rise and fall of the Catholic Church in modern Ireland*, 2nd edn (Dublin: UCD Press, 1998).

12. James M. Smith, *Ireland's Magdalen Laundries and the Nation's Architecture of Containment* (Manchester: Manchester University Press, 2007), pp. 5–20.

13. For an excellent analysis of the report, see Catriona Crowe, 'The Commission and the Survivors', *The Dublin Review*, no. 83, summer 2021, pp. 12–27.

14. Cited at Rosemary Hennessy, *Profit and Pleasure: Sexual identities in late capitalism* (London: Routledge, 2000), pp. 214–15.

15. Ibid., pp. 216–17.

16. Herbert Marcuse, *One-Dimensional Man* (London: Sphere Books, 1968), p. 72.

17. For a perceptive overview, see Susan McKay, 'How the "Rugby Rape Trial" Divided Ireland', *Guardian*, 4 December 2018, www.

theguardian.com/news/2018/dec/04/rugby-rape-trial-ireland-belfast-case.

18. Raymond Williams, *Marxism and Literature* (Oxford: Oxford University Press, 1977), pp. 95–100.

19. Walter Benjamin, 'Paris, Capital of the Nineteenth Century', in *The Arcades Project*, trans. Howard Eiland and Kevin McLaughlin (Cambridge, MA: Harvard University Press, 2002), pp. 14–26.

20. Lucas Ramon Mendos, *State-Sponsored Homophobia 2019* (Geneva: ILGA [International Lesbian, Gay, Bisexual, Trans and Intersex Association], 2019).

21. Two Fuse, *Freedom?*, pp. 51–5. See also Eilís Ward, *Self* (Cork: Cork University Press, 2021).

22. The image can be found at gcn.ie/magazine/love-equality.

23. Herbert Marcuse, *Eros and Civilisation* (New York: Vintage, 1962 [1955]), p. 86.

24. Cited at Katherine Sender, *Business, Not Politics: The making of the gay market* (New York: Columbia University Press, 2005), p. 13.

25. Ibid.

26. Ibid., p. 11.

27. Alderson, *Sex, Needs and Queer Culture*, p. 71.

28. Alison Shonkwiller, 'The Selfish-Enough Father: Gay adoption and the late capitalist family', *GLQ: A journal of lesbian and gay studies*, vol. 14, no. 4, 2008, pp. 537–67, at p. 550.

29. Alison Phipps, *Me, Not You: The trouble with mainstream feminism* (Manchester: Manchester University Press, 2020), p. 8.

30. For an incisive critique of the neoliberal and reformist underpinnings of the Irish marriage equality campaign, see Anne Mulhall, 'The Republic of Love', https://bullybloggers.wordpress.

com/2015/06/20/the-republic-of-love (20 June 2015), and Aidan Beatty, 'From Gay Power to Gay Rights', https://www. jacobinmag.com/2015/05/ireland-gay-marriage-referendum-rights-movement (29 May 2015).

31. Wendy Brown, *Edgework: Critical essays on knowledge and politics* (Princeton NJ: Princeton University Press, 2005), p. 3.

32. Melinda Cooper, *Family Values: Between neoliberalism and the new social conservatism* (New York: Zone Books, 2017), p. 209.

33. Ibid., p. 210.

34. Ibid., p. 214.

35. Love Equality is a campaigning organisation for marriage rights in Northern Ireland, where equal marriage came into law in January 2020.

36. Ronit Lentin, 'Ireland: Racial state and crisis racism', *Ethnic and Racial Studies*, vol. 30, no. 4, 2007, pp. 610–27.

37. Anne Mulhall, 'Queer in Ireland: Deviant filiations and the (un)holy family', in Lisa Downing and Robert Grillett (eds), *Queer in Europe* (Farnham: Ashgate, 2011), p. 101.

38. Ibid., p. 105.

39. Cited at ibid., p. 107.

40. Ibid.

41. Bulelani Mfaco, 'I Live in Direct Provision. It's a Devastating System – and It Has Thrown Away Millions', *Irish Times*, 4 July 2020. Mfaco is a journalist and a spokesperson for MASI (Movement of Asylum Seekers in Ireland).

42. See, for instance, Melatu Uche Okorie, *This Hostel Life* (Dublin: Skein Press, 2018).

43. Paul Ryan, *Male Sex Work in the Digital Age: Curated lives* (London: Palgrave Macmillan, 2019), p. 2.

44. Ibid., p. 42.

45. Ibid., pp. 8–9.

46. Finn Bowring, 'Repressive Desublimation and Consumer Culture: Re-evaluating Herbert Marcuse', *new formations*, no. 75, 2012, p. 12.

47. Marcuse, *Eros and Civilisation*, p. 40.

48. Wendy Brown, *Undoing the Demos: Neoliberalism's stealth revolution* (New York: Zone Books, 2015), pp. 35–45.

49. Jodi Dean, *Democracy and other Neoliberal Fantasies: Communicative capitalism and left politics* (Durham, NC: Duke University Press, 2009). For a useful overview of the political evolution of this concept, see Harry Brown, *Public Sphere* (Cork: Cork University Press, 2018), pp. 100–17.

50. Ryan, *Male Sex Work*, pp. 65–72.

51. Ibid., p. 77.

52. Ibid., pp. 105–8.

53. Una Mullally, *In the Name of Love: The movement for marriage equality in Ireland. An oral history* (Dublin: History Press Ireland, 2014), pp. 97–106, 150–9; Sonja Tiernan, *The History of Marriage Equality in Ireland: A social revolution begins* (Manchester: Manchester University Press, 2020), p. 61.

54. Mullally, *In the Name of Love*, 'Introduction' and p. 1.

55. 'The Road to Marriage Equality: Remembering Declan Flynn', *Hot Press*, 22 May 2020, hotpress.com/culture/road-marriage-equality-remembering-declan-flynn-22816207. The original article was by Joseph Healey.

56. Ger Philpott, 'Declan Flynn: The Fairview murder that ignited the Irish pride movement', *GCN*, 26 June 2020, gcn.ie/declan-flynn-fairview-park-murder-pride; Lauren Heskin, 'The Murder of Declan Flynn and the History of Dublin Pride', *Image*, 24 June

2020, image.ie/life/declan-flynn-fairview-park-dublin-pride-history-205273.

57. My concern here echoes that of his family, who believe that the contemporary memorialisation risks effacing Declan's vitality and kindness. See Simon Carswell, 'Declan Flynn "Queerbashing" Murder "Still Very Raw" 36 Years On', *Irish Times*, 30 June 2018.

58. Judith Butler, *Precarious Life: The powers of mourning and politics* (London: Verso, 2004), p. 22.

59. Ibid., p. 30.

60. Wendy Brown, *States of Injury: Power and freedom in late modernity* (Princeton, NJ: Princeton University Press, 1996), p. 54.

61. Ibid., p. 69.

62. For an insightful Marxist-feminist analysis of that campaign, see Sinéad Kennedy, 'Ireland's Fight for Choice', *Jacobin*, 25 March 2018, https://www.jacobinmag.com/2018/03/irelands-fight-for-choice. See also Sinéad Kennedy, '"#Repealthe8th": Ireland, abortion access and the movement to remove the eighth amendment', *Anthropologia*, vol. 5, no. 2, 2018, pp. 13–31, https://mural.maynoothuniversity.ie/12936.

63. Butler, *Precarious Life*, pp. 26–7.

64. Ibid., p. 26.

65. Judith Butler, *The Force of Non-Violence* (London: Verso, 2020), p. 41.

66. Ibid., p. 42.

67. For further exploration of this idea, see Ward, *Self*.

68. Butler, *Precarious Life*, p. 27.

69. This description and manifesto for the production can be found at: anuproductions.ie/work/faultline-2019.

70. Herbert O. Mackey (ed.), *The Crime Against Europe: The writings and poetry of Roger Casement* (Dublin: C.J. Fallon, 1958), p. 170.

71. Declan Kiberd, *Inventing Ireland* (London: Vintage, 1996), pp. 136–54.

72. For a useful critique of 'progressivism' in political and historical thought, see Laird, *Commemoration*, pp. 38–46.

73. Michelle O Riordan, *The Gaelic Mind and the Collapse of the Gaelic World* (Cork: Cork University Press, 1990), pp. 250–5.

74. John P. Harrington, *Modern and Contemporary Irish Drama*, 2nd edn (New York: W.W. Norton, 2009), p. 351. Ellipsis in original.

75. James Penney, *After Queer Theory: The limits of sexual politics* (London: Pluto Press, 2014), p. 6.

76. Angus Mitchell, *16 Lives: Roger Casement* (Dublin: O'Brien Press, 2013), pp. 352–3.

77. Rob Nixon, *Slow Violence and the Environmentalism of the Poor* (Cambridge, MA: Harvard University Press, 2011), p. 41.

78. Ibid., p. 2.

79. Ibid., p. 15.

80. Séamas Ó Síocháin and Michael O'Sullivan (eds), *The Eyes of Another Race: Roger Casement's Congo report and 1903 diary* (Dublin: UCD Press, 2003), p. 53.

81. Adam Hochschild, *King Leopold's Ghost: A story of greed, terror and heroism in colonial Africa* (London: Macmillan, 1999), p. 165.

82. Ó Síocháin and O'Sullivan (eds), *The Eyes of Another Race*, p. 72.

83. Ibid., p. 15.

84. Angus Mitchell (ed.), *The Amazon Journal of Roger Casement* (Dublin: Lilliput Press, 1997), pp. 133, 151.

85. Ibid., pp. 144, 198.

86. Ó Síocháin and O'Sullivan (eds), *The Eyes of Another Race*, p. 53.

87. Ibid., pp. 196–207.

88. Ibid., p. 202.

89. Alan Sinfield, *On Sexuality and Power* (New York: Columbia University Press, 2004), p. 73.

90. Roger Sawyer (ed.), *Roger Casement's Diaries 1910: The black and the white* (London: Pimlico, 1997), p. 51.

91. Ibid., p. 44.

92. Margaret O'Callaghan and Angus Mitchell provide a cogent analysis of the complex, evolving and productive relationship between Casement's nationalist and internationalist politics. See Margaret O'Callaghan, '"With the Eyes of Another Race, of a People once Hunted Themselves": Casement, colonialism and a remembered past', in Mary E. Daly (ed.), *Roger Casement in Irish and World History* (Dublin: Royal Irish Academy, 2005), and Mitchell, *16 Lives*, pp. 154–72.

93. Simon Fujiwara, *The Humanizer*, and Alan Phelan, *Our Kind*; the latter was installed in Dublin's Hugh Lane Gallery as part of an exhibition based around *High Treason*, John Lavery's famous painting of Casement's trial. *Butterflies and Bones*, choreographed by Fearghus Ó Conchúir. *The Casement Sonata*, composed by Gavin Friday.

94. Martin Mansergh, 'Roger Casement and the Idea of a Broader Nationalist Tradition: His impact on Anglo-Irish relations', in Mary E. Daly (ed.), *Roger Casement in Irish and World History* (Dublin: Royal Irish Academy, 2005), p. 189.

95. Colm Tóibín, *Love in a Dark Time: Gay lives from Wilde to Almodóvar* (London: Picador, 2001), p. 105.

96. Fiona Loughnane, '"With the Eyes of Another Race": Congo atrocity photographs and the commemoration of Easter 1916',

Review of Irish Studies in Europe, vol. 2, no. 2, 2018, pp. 19–39, at p. 20. For a critical overview of the broader context within which the Casement events took place, officially known as the Decade of Centenaries, along with a searching examination of the conservative or radical potential of such commemorative activity, see Laird, *Commemoration*.

97. It is worth noting the complexity of views here. Angus Mitchell argues that the diaries *were* forged by British intelligence agents, but he does so from an avowedly anti-homophobic and gay-affirmative perspective.

98. From the late 1970s until 2008 the Irish Queer Archive was managed by the National Gay Federation (NGF, later the National Lesbian and Gay Federation, NLGF, and currently known as NFX). Since 2008 the archive has been held and managed by the National Library of Ireland in Dublin. This photograph illustrated an article in *The Irish Times* in June 2013 and can be seen here: www.irishtimes.com/life-and-style/people/three-decades-of-pride–1.1438646.

99. Patrick McDonagh, '"Homosexuals Are Revolting": Gay and lesbian activism in the Republic of Ireland 1970s–1990s', *Studi irlandesi: A journal of Irish studies*, no. 7, 2017, pp. 65–91. See also *Gay and Lesbian Activism in the Republic of Ireland, 1973–93* (London: Bloomsbury, 2021). Maurice Casey, 'Radical Politics and Gay Activism in the Republic of Ireland, 1974–1990', *Irish Studies Review*, vol. 26, no. 2, 2018, pp. 217–36.

100. McDonagh, '"Homosexuals Are Revolting"', p. 68.

101. Cited at Casey, 'Radical Politics', p. 220.

102. Ibid., p. 222.

103. For an informative and lively account of this march, see McDonagh, '"Homosexuals Are Revolting"', pp. 83–6.

104. Mick Quinlan, 'Some Class of a Scene', in *Out for Ourselves: The lives of Irish lesbians and gay men* (Dublin: Dublin Lesbian and

Gay Men's Collective and Women's Press, 1986), pp. 84–6. This collection was collaboratively edited by DLGC members.

105. Dennis Altman, *Homosexual: Oppression and liberation* (London: Serpent's Tail, 1971), p. 241.

106. Kieran Rose, *Diverse Communities: The evolution of lesbian and gay politics in Ireland* (Cork: Cork University Press, 1993), p. 2.

107. Ibid., p. 3.

108. Ibid.

109. Peadar Kirby, 'Contested Pedigrees of the Celtic Tiger', in Peadar Kirby, Luke Gibbons and Michael Cronin (eds), *Reinventing Ireland: Culture, society and the global economy* (London: Pluto, 2001), p. 32. See also the essays by Colin Coulter, Denis O'Hearn and Kieran Allen in Colin Coulter and Steve Coleman (eds), *The End of Irish History? Critical approaches to the 'Celtic Tiger'* (Manchester: Manchester University Press, 2001).

110. For a detailed analysis of the operation, scale and destination of this wealth redistribution, see Kieran Allen, *The Celtic Tiger: The myth of social partnership in Ireland* (Manchester: Manchester University Press, 2000), pp. 59–77.

111. Casey, 'Radical Politics', pp. 28–30.

112. Marcuse, *Eros and Civilisation*, p. 44.

113. Ibid., p. 184.

114. Una Mullally, 'Joe Caslin Installs Second Mural on the Side of a Castle', *Irish Times*, 19 May 2015, https://www.irishtimes.com/news/ireland/irish-news/joe-caslin-installs-second-mural-on-the-side-of-a-castle-1.2218016; Oisin Kenny, 'Conversations in Monochrome' (October 2019), www.gcn.ie/magazine/love-equality; 'Joe Caslin's New Mural Gets Pride of Place in Belfast', *GCN*, 3 August 2016, https://gcn.ie/joe-caslins-new-mural-gets-pride-place-belfast.

115. Peter Corboy, 'Interview with Joe Caslin' (29 June 2017), https://www.designboom.com/art/joe-caslin-interview-irish-street-art-06-29-2017.

116. The video can be viewed at www.joecaslin.com.

117. The details are available on the National Museum of Ireland website. See 'Giant Mural Shining a Spotlight on Mental Health', https://www.thejournal.ie/mental-health-mural-national-museum-3594543-Sep2017/.

118. Eimear Sparks, 'Joe Caslin – Interview', www.thebridgetcd.com/2016/02/02/joe-caslin.

119. For details on the project, see 'Finding Power, by Joe Caslin' on the National Gallery of Ireland website at www.nationalgallery.ie/finding-power-joe-caslin.

120. Walter Benjamin, 'Theses on the Philosophy of History', in *Illuminations*, trans. Harry Zohn, ed. Hannah Arendt (New York: Shocken Books, 2007 [1969]), p. 255.

121. Henri Lefebvre, *The Production of Space*, trans. Donald Nicholson-Smith (London: Blackwell 1991 [1974]), p. 165.

122. Ibid., p. 166.

123. Butler, *Force of Non-Violence*, p. 49.

124. For further exploration of this idea, see Ward, *Self*.

125. Ernst Bloch, *The Principle of Hope*, vol. 3, trans. Neville Plaice, Stephen Plaice and Paul Knight (Cambridge, MA: MIT Press, 1986), p. 197. (Original German-language publication, 1959.)

126. Ibid., p. 932.

127. Ibid., vol. 1, pp. 246, 196.

128. Marcuse, *Eros and Civilisation*, pp. 131–2.

129. Ibid., p. 63. Here Marcuse redefines *Agape* – commonly understood as 'Christian' love, distinct from erotic or sexual love – as a version of his conception of Eros; that is, a form of love in which that distinction between the erotic and non-erotic has ceased to be meaningful.

130. Ibid., pp. 63–4.

131. Ibid., p. 153.

132. Ibid., p. 45.

133. In January 2014 Rory O'Neill, creator of Panti Bliss, was interviewed on RTÉ television. Subsequently, a group of right-wing journalists, including John Waters, Breda O'Brien and David Quinn, along with others associated with the Iona Institute, a reactionary Catholic lobbying group, threatened legal proceedings against the state broadcaster claiming that O'Neill had defamed them by describing their work as homophobic. Without challenging their claim, RTÉ promptly broadcast an apology and paid the group €85,000 as 'compensation'.

134. Emer O'Toole, 'Guerrilla Glamour: The queer tactics of Dr Panti Bliss', *Éire-Ireland*, vol. 52, nos. 3 & 4, 2018, pp. 104–21, at p. 117.

135. Judith Butler, *Gender Trouble: Feminism and the subversion of identity* (London: Routledge, 1990), pp. 1–34.

136. Marcuse, *Eros and Civilisation*, p. 118.

Bibliography

(All URLs are valid at time of going to press)

Alderson, David, *Sex, Needs and Queer Culture: From liberation to the post-gay* (London: Zed Books, 2016)

Allen, Kieran, *The Celtic Tiger: The myth of social partnership in Ireland* (Manchester: Manchester University Press, 2000)

Altman, Dennis, *Homosexual: Oppression and liberation* (London: Serpent's Tail, 1971)

Bardon, Sarah, 'Varadkar Wants to Lead Party for "People Who Get Up Early in the Morning"', *Irish Times*, 20 May 2017, https://www.irishtimes.com/news/politics/varadkar-wants-to-lead-party-for-people-who-get-up-early-in-the-morning-1.3090753

Beatty, Aidan, 'From Gay Power to Gay Rights', *Jacobin*, 29 May 2015

Benjamin, Walter, *The Arcades Project*, trans. Howard Eiland and Kevin McLaughlin (Cambridge, MA: Harvard University Press, 2002)

—, *Illuminations*, trans. Harry Zohn, ed. Hannah Arendt (New York: Shocken Books, 2007)

Bloch, Ernst, *The Principle of Hope* (3 volumes), vol. 3, trans. Neville Plaice, Stephen Plaice and Paul Knight (Cambridge, MA: MIT Press, 1986)

Bowring, Finn, 'Repressive Desublimation and Consumer Culture: Re-evaluating Herbert Marcuse', *new formations*, no. 75, 2012

Brown, Harry, *Public Sphere* (Cork: Cork University Press, 2018)

Brown, Wendy, *States of Injury: Power and freedom in late modernity* (Princeton, NJ: Princeton University Press, 1996)

—, *Edgework: Critical essays on knowledge and politics* (Princeton, NJ: Princeton University Press, 2005)

—, 'American Nightmare: Neoliberalism, neoconservatism, and de-democratisation', *Political Theory*, vol. 34, no. 6, 2006

—, *Undoing the Demos: Neoliberalism's stealth revolution* (New York: Zone Books, 2015)

Butler, Judith, *Gender Trouble: Feminism and the subversion of identity* (London: Routledge, 1990)

—, *Precarious Life: The powers of mourning and politics* (London: Verso, 2004)

—, *The Force of Non-Violence* (London: Verso, 2020)

Carswell, Simon, 'Declan Flynn "Queerbashing" Murder "Still Very Raw" 36 Years On', *Irish Times*, 30 June 2018

Casey, Maurice, 'Radical Politics and Gay Activism in the Republic of Ireland, 1974–1990', *Irish Studies Review*, vol. 26, no. 2, 2018

Cooper, Melinda, *Family Values: Between neoliberalism and the new social conservatism* (New York: Zone Books, 2017)

Corboy, Peter, 'Interview with Joe Caslin' (29 June 2017), https://www.designboom.com/art/joe-caslin-interview-irish-street-art-06-29-2017

Coulter, Colin and Steve Coleman (eds), *The End of Irish History? Critical approaches to the 'Celtic Tiger'* (Manchester: Manchester University Press, 2001)

Crowe, Catriona, 'The Commission and the Survivors', *The Dublin Review*, no. 83, summer 2021

Dean, Jodi, *Democracy and other Neoliberal Fantasies: Communicative capitalism and left politics* (Durham, NC: Duke University Press, 2009)

Finnegan, Brian, 'The Varadkar Paradox', *GCN*, no. 332, August 2017, https://pocketmags.com/eu/gcn-magazine/332/articles/179754/the-varadkar-paradox

Harrington, John P., *Modern and Contemporary Irish Drama*, 2nd edn (New York: W.W. Norton, 2009)

Hennessy, Rosemary, *Profit and Pleasure: Sexual identities in late capitalism* (London: Routledge, 2000)

Heskin, Lauren, 'The Murder of Declan Flynn and the History of Dublin Pride', *Image*, 24 June 2020, image.ie/life/declan-flynn-fairview-park-dublin-pride-history-205273

Hochschild, Adam, *King Leopold's Ghost: A story of greed, terror and heroism in colonial Africa* (London: Macmillan, 1999)

Inglis, Tom, *Moral Monopoly: The rise and fall of the Catholic Church in modern Ireland*, 2nd edn (Dublin: UCD Press, 1998)

Kennedy, Sinéad, 'Ireland's Fight for Choice', *Jacobin*, 25 March 2018, https://www.jacobinmag.com/2018/03/irelands-fight-for-choice.

—, '"#Repealthe8th": Ireland, abortion access and the movement to remove the eighth amendment', *Anthropologia*, vol. 5, no. 2, 2018, pp. 13–31, https://mural.maynoothuniversity.ie/12936

Kenny, Oisin, 'Conversations in Monochrome' (October 2019), www.gcn.ie/magazine/love-equality.

Kerrigan, Páraic and Maria Pramaggiore, 'Homoheroic or Homophobic? Leo Varadkar, LGBTQ politics and contemporary news narratives', *Critical Studies in Media Communication*, vol. 38, no. 2, 2021

Kiberd, Declan, *Inventing Ireland* (London: Vintage, 1996)

Kirby, Peadar, Luke Gibbons and Michael Cronin (eds), *Reinventing Ireland: Culture, society and the global economy* (London: Pluto, 2001)

Laird, Heather, *Commemoration* (Cork: Cork University Press, 2018)

Lefebvre, Henri, *The Production of Space*, trans. Donald Nicholson-Smith (London: Blackwell, 1991)

Lentin, Ronit, 'Ireland: Racial state and crisis racism', *Ethnic and Racial Studies*, vol. 30, no. 4, 2007

Loughnane, Fiona, '"With the Eyes of Another Race": Congo atrocity photographs and the commemoration of Easter 1916', *Review of Irish Studies in Europe*, vol. 2, no. 2, 2018

MacCarthy, Anna and Aoife O'Driscoll, 'Leo Varadkar Will Be as Helpful to the Gays as Margaret Thatcher Was to Women', *GCN*, 6 June 2017, https://gcn.ie/leo-varadkar-margaret-thatcher

Mackey, Herbert O. (ed.), *The Crime Against Europe: The writings and poetry of Roger Casement* (Dublin: C.J. Fallon, 1958)

Mansergh, Martin, 'Roger Casement and the Idea of a Broader Nationalist Tradition: His impact on Anglo-Irish relations', in Mary E. Daly (ed.), *Roger Casement in Irish and World History* (Dublin: Royal Irish Academy, 2005)

Marcuse, Herbert, *Eros and Civilisation* (New York: Vintage, 1962)

—, *One-Dimensional Man* (London: Sphere Books, 1968)

McDonagh, Patrick, '"Homosexuals Are Revolting": Gay and lesbian activism in the Republic of Ireland 1970s–1990s', *Studi irlandesi: A journal of Irish studies*, no. 7, 2017

—, *Gay and Lesbian Activism in the Republic of Ireland, 1973–93* (London: Bloomsbury, 2021)

McKay, Susan, 'How the "Rugby Rape Trial" Divided Ireland', *Guardian*, 4 December 2018, www.theguardian.com/news/2018/dec/04/rugby-rape-trial-ireland-belfast-case

Mendos, Lucas Ramon, *State-Sponsored Homophobia 2019* (Geneva: ILGA [International Lesbian, Gay, Bisexual, Trans and Intersex Association], 2019)

Mfaco, Bulelani, 'I Live in Direct Provision. It's a Devastating System – and It Has Thrown Away Millions', *Irish Times*, 4 July 2020

Mitchell, Angus (ed.), *The Amazon Journal of Roger Casement* (Dublin: Lilliput Press, 1997)

—, *16 Lives: Roger Casement* (Dublin: O'Brien Press, 2013)

Mulhall, Anne, 'Queer in Ireland: Deviant filiations and the (un)holy family', in Lisa Downing and Robert Grillett (eds), *Queer in Europe* (Farnham: Ashgate, 2011), p. 101

—, 'The Republic of Love' (20 June 2015), https://bullybloggers.wordpress.com/2015/06/20/the-republic-of-love

Mullally, Una, *In The Name of Love: the movement for marriage equality in Ireland, an oral history* (Dublin: History Press Ireland, 2014)

—, 'Joe Caslin Installs Second Mural on the Side of a Castle', *Irish Times*, 19 May 2015, https://www.irishtimes.com/news/ireland/irish-news/joe-caslin-installs-second-mural-on-the-side-of-a-castle-1.2218016

—, 'Varadkar Election a Strange One for LGBT People', *Irish Times*, 5 June 2017, https://www.irishtimes.com/opinion/varadkar-election-a-strange-one-for-lgbt-people-1.3107615

Nixon, Rob, *Slow Violence and the Environmentalism of the Poor* (Cambridge, MA: Harvard University Press, 2011)

O'Callaghan, Margaret, '"With the Eyes of Another Race, of a People once Hunted Themselves": Casement, colonialism and a remembered past', in Mary E. Daly (ed.), *Roger Casement in Irish and World History* (Dublin: Royal Irish Academy, 2005)

Okorie, Melatu Uche, *This Hostel Life* (Dublin: Skein Press, 2018)

O Riordan, Michelle, *The Gaelic Mind and the Collapse of the Gaelic World* (Cork: Cork University Press, 1990)

Ó Síocháin, Séamas and Michael O'Sullivan (eds), *The Eyes of Another Race: Roger Casement's Congo report and 1903 diary* (Dublin: UCD Press, 2003)

O'Toole, Emer, 'Guerrilla Glamour: The queer tactics of Dr Panti Bliss', *Éire-Ireland*, vol. 52, nos. 3 & 4, 2018

Penney, James, *After Queer Theory: The limits of sexual politics* (London: Pluto Press, 2014)

Philpott, Ger, 'Declan Flynn: The Fairview murder that ignited the Irish pride movement', *GCN*, 26 June 2020, gcn.ie/declan-flynn-fairview-park-murder-pride

Phipps, Alison, *Me, Not You: The trouble with mainstream feminism* (Manchester: Manchester University Press, 2020)

Quinlan, Mick, 'Some Class of a Scene', in *Out for Ourselves: The lives of Irish lesbians and gay men* (Dublin: Dublin Lesbian and Gay Men's Collective and Women's Press, 1986)

Rose, Kieran, *Diverse Communities: The evolution of lesbian and gay politics in Ireland* (Cork: Cork University Press, 1993)

Ryan, Paul, *Male Sex Work in the Digital Age: Curated lives* (London: Palgrave Macmillan, 2019)

Sawyer, Roger (ed.), *Roger Casement's Diaries 1910: The black and the white* (London: Pimlico, 1997)

Sender, Katherine, *Business, Not Politics: The making of the gay market* (New York: Columbia University Press, 2005)

Shonkwiller, Alison, 'The Selfish-Enough Father: Gay adoption and the late capitalist family', *GLQ: A journal of lesbian and gay studies*, vol. 14, no. 4, 2008

Sinfield, Alan, *On Sexuality and Power* (New York: Columbia University Press, 2004)

Smith, James M., *Ireland's Magdalen Laundries and the Nation's Architecture of Containment* (Manchester: Manchester University Press, 2007)

Tiernan, Sonja, *The History of Marriage Equality in Ireland: A social revolution begins* (Manchester: Manchester University Press, 2020)

Tóibín, Colm, *Love in a Dark Time: Gay lives from Wilde to Almodóvar* (London: Picador, 2001)

Two Fuse, *Freedom?* (Cork: Cork University Press, 2018)

Ward, Eilís, *Self* (Cork: Cork University Press, 2021)

Williams, Raymond, *Marxism and Literature* (Oxford: Oxford University Press, 1977)

Index

abjection, 46, 56

abortion, 3, 13, 14, 33, 59, 96, 98

abortion referendums, 33, 59, 98

ACT-UP, 30

advertising, 8, 19, 24–7, 42, 45

affirmation, 23, 29, 49, 63–4, 66–7

affluence, 5, 10, 24, 26; *see also* wealth

Afghanistan, 54

AIDS, 30–31, 107–8

Alderson, David, 2, 27

alienation, 18, 41, 57, 61, 64, 98

Altman, Dennis, 100

anger, 51–2, 56

anti-capitalism, 9, 57, 84–5, 89, 103, 130

anti-colonialism, 19, 84, 86–7, 88, 95, 99, 103, 121

anti-imperialism, 9, 55, 84, 86, 89, 96, 102

ANU, 61–7

appropriated space, 118

'Ar Scáth a Chéile a Mhaireann na Daoine' (Caslin), 112–13, 119

Arnold, Matthew, 70

art, 11, 19, 84, 89–90, 111–23, 128–30

assimilation, 63, 95, 100, 104, 108

asylum process, 36–7, 85

Auden, W.H., 89

autonomy, 4, 13, 24, 29, 59, 118, 120

Banna Strand, 86

Beatty, Aidan, 49

Belfast, 111

Benjamin, Walter, 22, 117

Bhebe, Nanci, 63–4

bio-politics, 33, 34, 36

Bloch, Ernst, 10–11, 73, 120, 121–2

Bowring, Finn, 41

Brecht, Bertolt, 64

Brehon Laws, 102

Brown, Wendy, 3–4, 9, 30, 42, 55–8

Buenos Aires, 83

Burke, Thomas, 83

Burton, Frederic William, 116

Butler, Judith, 8, 54–5, 58–61, 119, 127

Butterflies and Bones (Ó Conchúir), 90

Caher Castle, 111

capitalism, 5–11, 13–23, 25, 27, 29, 40–41, 46, 55–8, 61, 71, 74–6, 79–85, 89–91, 97, 99–101, 109, 110, 118, 123, 125, 128

Casement, Roger, 9–10, 69–91, 94–5, 125

Casey, Maurice, 96–7, 98, 106–7

Caslin, Joe, 11, 111–23, 125, 128–30

Catholic Church, 15–16, 107

Catholicism, 1, 13–16, 35, 88, 89, 107

Cavendish, Lord Frederick, 83

censorship, 127

child sexual abuse, 15

Christ, 123

citizenship, 4, 32–6, 46

citizenship referendum, 32–6

citoyen, 120–21

civil partnerships, 31, 34, 50

civil rights, 100

'Claddagh Embrace, The' (Caslin), 111, 112, 116, 125, 127, 129

class, 5, 38, 43, 58, 98, 99, 100, 106, 119, 128

climate change, 56

Clinton, Bill, 31

Coffey, Cormac, 115

collectivism, 2, 11, 27, 28, 64

Collins Barracks, 114–16

colonialism, 19, 25, 73–5, 76–80, 83–4, 86–7, 102

commemoration, 9–10, 53, 68, 84, 86–91, 94–5

commodification, 11, 17, 26, 38, 42, 82

communication technologies, 83

communicative capitalism, 43, 75

community, 36, 39, 54, 59–61

Congo, 73, 76–80, 81, 83

Connolly, James, 84, 88

conservative nationalism, 14, 15

Constitution of Ireland, 14, 21, 59, 98

consumerism, 4, 7, 22, 30

containment, 14–15

contraception, 13, 14

Cooper, Melinda, 30–31

Cork, 51, 96, 103

cosmopolitanism, 23, 35

criminalisation, 14, 50–51, 94, 113–14; *see also* decriminalisation

crucifixion imagery, 121, 123

cruising, 51, 66–7, 74, 81–2, 88–9, 91, 125

cultural nationalism, 69–71, 88

dance, 24, 65–7, 84, 90

Dean, Jodi, 43

decriminalisation, 96, 97–8, 101–3, 104, 107; *see also* criminalisation

Defence Forces, 94

democracy, 4, 7, 19, 23, 105

dependency, 29, 54, 60–61, 68, 119, 120

desire, 16, 18–19, 44, 72–4, 87–8, 100, 109

direct provision, 36–8, 113

disability, 35, 59, 116

Diverse Communities (Rose), 101–4, 108

diversity, 2, 6, 35, 85, 89, 126

divorce, 13, 14, 107

divorce referendum, 107

domestic labour, 17, 28

dominated space, 118

domination, 20, 41, 118, 123

Douglas, Alfred, 72

drag performers, 52, 116, 126

drug use, 113–14

Dublin, 9, 10, 21, 33, 34–5, 38–9, 51–3, 61–2, 82–3, 88, 93–6, 103, 111, 113–16

Dublin Lesbian and Gay Collective (DLGC), 10, 95–6, 98–9, 110

Dublin Lesbian and Gay Film Festival, 34–5

DublinLive website, 52

Easter Rising, 84, 88, 94–5, 114

Edinburgh, 112

education, 42, 46, 88

eighth amendment, 3, 59

Ekulite, Mola, 78

emigration, 63, 107

entrepreneurism, 10, 24, 28, 42, 56, 120

environment, 56, 75–6

equality, 7, 8, 29–32, 35, 38, 45–50, 103–4, 106, 129

Equality Authority, 104

Eros, 18–19, 109–10, 122–5

European Court of Human Rights, 96, 102

exclusion, 35–6, 57–8, 97, 98

exploitation, 9, 23, 33, 39, 57, 61, 73, 82

expressionism, 117

Fairview Park, 51–2, 99

family, 5, 27–8, 30–31, 100, 109, 126

fantasy, 73, 83, 122, 125

Faultline (ANU), 61–7

feminism, 2, 6, 13–14, 19, 52, 55, 58–9, 98, 99, 107

Ferguson, Ann, 16

Fianna Fáil, 85

financialisation, 2, 56

'Finding Power' (Caslin), 116, 119

flogging, 78–9

Flynn, Declan, 9, 51–4, 65, 68, 98

Fornoff, Erin, 114

freedom, 7, 13, 16–20, 29, 38, 43, 56, 97, 100–101

Freud, Sigmund, 40, 109, 124–5

Friel, Brian, 71

Galway, 96

gambling, 81, 91

gardaí, 51, 62, 65, 93–5

Gate Theatre, 61

Gay and Lesbian Equality Network (GLEN), 103–4, 106

Gay Defence Committee, 96

Gay Pride, 51, 53, 93–5

Gays Against Imperialism, 96

Gays Against the Amendment, 96, 98

GCN, 3, 4–5, 6, 24–8, 31–2, 36, 38, 52, 53, 86

gender roles, 17, 28

General Post Office (GPO), 94–5

gig economy, 43

globalisation, 2, 19, 105

grief, 10, 52, 54–5

Grindr, 41

guiding images, 11, 120, 130

gyms, 39, 42, 44, 46

Hall, Stuart, 25

happiness, 26, 38

healthcare, 30–31, 46

Healy, Gráinne, 48

hegemony, 7, 13, 15, 23, 89, 118, 120, 128

'Hellelil and Hildebrand' (Burton), 116

Hennessy, Rosemary, 16–17

heterosexuality, 35, 58, 100, 126

History of Marriage Equality in Ireland, The (Tiernan), 48–50

Hochschild, Adam, 77–8, 84

homoeroticism, 8, 72

homoheroism, 2–3, 4, 6, 10, 23–4

homophobia, 2–3, 5, 8, 9, 23, 55–6, 58, 66–7, 88, 102, 107, 126, 129

hope, 10–11, 38, 73, 121–2, 129–30

Hot Press, 52, 53

housing, 15, 26, 37, 39, 46

human body, 59–61, 66–7, 74–82, 87–8, 90–91, 107–10, 118–20, 122–4; *see also* male body

human rights, 36, 37, 102

Hyde, Douglas, 69

identity, 5–6, 9–10, 17, 25–6, 55–9, 67, 68, 71–2, 87–90, 100, 102, 108, 126–7

Image, 52, 53

imagination, 9, 19, 73, 122

In the Name of Love (Mullally), 47–8, 50–52

inceldom, 58

inclusion, 29, 31, 55–6, 57–8

individualism, 2, 9, 11, 27, 28, 60, 64, 97

industrial schools, 14

inequality, 8, 32, 46, 106, 129

injury, 9, 55–6, 61–8, 90–91, 108, 129

Instagram, 41, 44

instrumentalism, 71, 82

interdependence, 28, 60–61

internationalism, 84, 88

intimacy, 8, 11, 16, 45, 64, 66, 67, 109, 125

Iraq, 54

Ireland Says Yes (Healy, Sheehan & Whelan), 48

IrishCentral website, 52

Irish Council for Civil Liberties, 103

Irish Free State, 14

Irish Gay Rights Movement (IGRM), 20, 61–2, 97

Irish language, 69–72

Irish Queer Archive, 62, 93

Keogh, Rachael, 114

Kerrigan, Cathal, 99

Kerrigan, Páraic, 1–3

Kirby, Peadar, 105

labour, 3, 17, 28, 39, 41, 43, 45–6, 61, 104, 105, 109–10, 121

law, 14, 27, 50–51, 94, 97–8, 102–3, 107

Law Reform Commission, 103

Lefebvre, Henri, 118

Lentin, Ronit, 33

LGBT movement, 3, 6, 10, 13–14, 20, 30–31, 34–5, 50–53, 55, 58–9, 61–3, 65, 93–108

liberation, 7–8, 10, 11, 16–20, 63, 99–100, 110, 122–3, 125

Loughnane, Fiona, 86

love, 16, 29–30, 31–2

McDonagh, Patrick, 96

McDowell, Michael, 33, 34–5

Madeira, 80–81, 82

Magdalene asylums, 14

male body, 8, 9, 11, 39–43, 45–6, 66–7, 74, 81–2, 87–8, 90–91, 118–20, 122–4

Malone, Matthew, 65

Mansergh, Martin, 85

Marcuse, Herbert, 10, 18–20, 25, 40–41, 99, 109–10, 122–5

market economy, 3, 4, 26, 28, 37–8, 85, 106

marriage, 4, 8, 13, 18, 21, 24–38, 45, 47–50, 57, 67, 96, 100, 108–9, 111, 125–7, 129

marriage equality referendum, 21, 29–30, 32–6, 45, 47–50, 53, 86, 96, 108, 111, 125–7

Marx, Karl, 120

Marxism, 19, 63, 88, 99, 105

masculinism, 58, 98

media, 1–2, 34–5, 49, 52–3, 75, 84, 96, 97–8, 103–4, 111, 112, 117, 126

memorialisation see commemoration

memory, 83, 84, 117

mental health, 112–13, 115

Mfaco, Bulelani, 37

migrants, 33, 35–8

Minogue, Kylie, 2, 5

minoritarianism, 5, 57, 63, 68, 101, 106, 108, 128–9

misogyny, 2, 20, 58

Mitchell, Angus, 74, 84

mobilisation, 2, 7, 8–9, 10, 16, 23, 48, 52–3, 58–9, 63, 65, 96–101, 108

modernisation, 1, 34, 70, 110

Moloney, Stephen, 116, 119, 123

monetisation, 11, 26, 38, 42, 44–5

morality, 13, 15, 27, 106, 109, 110

Morris, Matthew, 90

mother and baby homes, 14–15

mourning, 54, 68

Mulhall, Anne, 33, 34, 35, 49

Mullally, Una, 47–8, 50–52, 108

murder, 51–4, 62, 65, 68, 96, 98

music, 2, 84

mutilation, 77–9

Narcissus, 123–4

National Gallery of Ireland, 116, 119, 123

National Gay Federation (NGF), 97–8, 99

National Museum of Ireland, 114–16

nationalism, 14, 15–16, 23, 34, 35, 58, 69–71, 83–4, 88, 89, 121

neoconservatism, 3–4, 31

neoliberalism, 2–4, 7, 8, 10–11, 16, 21–31, 36–8, 42–3, 46, 56, 75, 85, 89, 97, 105–6, 120, 126, 128

neutrality, 85

New Left, 99

New York Post, 1

Ní Chiarain, Ally, 114

Nietzsche, Friedrich, 56

9/11 attacks, 54

Nixon, Rob, 75–6

Norris, David, 50–51, 96, 102

Northern Ireland, 32, 111

O'Callaghan, Margaret, 84

O'Callaghan, Miriam, 1

Ó Conchúir, Fearghus, 90

O'Connell, Daniel, 70

O'Connell Street, 10, 93–5

O'Connor, Michael, 51

'On the Necesssity of De-Anglicising Ireland' (Hyde), 69

O'Neill, Rory, 52, 126–9

Onlyfans, 44

oppression, 13, 14, 16, 52, 53, 57, 66, 97, 99–101, 103, 127–8

oral history, 47

O'Reilly, Fiona, 114

Orpheus, 123

Ó Síocháin, Séamus, 78, 84

O'Sullivan, Michael, 78, 84

O'Toole, Emer, 126–8

'Our Nation's Sons' (Caslin), 112, 119, 128

outlawed needs, 17, 28

outsourcing, 37, 56

pain, 66, 74, 77–81, 91

Panti Bliss, 52, 126–9

partition, 14

patriarchy, 5, 29, 58, 100, 109

Pearse, Patrick, 84, 88

Penney, James, 72–3

Pentonville Prison, 90

performance principle, 40–41, 109, 120, 125

perversity, 124–5

Phipps, Alison, 28

pleasure, 9, 14, 16–19, 27, 28, 44, 45, 64, 66, 67, 74, 80–84, 87–8, 91, 109–10

pleasure principle, 41, 125

pluralism, 2, 29–30, 34, 35, 85, 89, 95, 104

Police Service of Northern Ireland (PSNI), 94

politicised identity, 55–8

pornography, 19–20, 44

power, 45–6, 56, 75, 85, 105, 117–18, 128–9

Pramaggiore, Maria, 1–3

precarity, 3, 39, 42, 43, 45

privatisation, 27–8, 37–8

profit, 7, 17, 19, 25, 26, 37–8, 42, 105

Programme for National Recovery, 104

progress, 49, 53, 70, 80, 110

property rights, 4, 15, 27, 29, 100

protest, 35, 51–2; *see also* mobilisation

Protestantism, 88

psychoanalysis, 123–4

Putumayo, 73, 80, 82, 83

queer theory, 126–7

Quinn, Stephen, 65–7

race, 33, 35, 37, 40, 58, 59, 64, 100

racialisation, 40

racism, 33, 35, 37, 58, 64

rape, 20

recession, 106–7

recognition, 36, 52, 55–6, 64–5, 67, 68, 96, 99, 100, 126, 129

reformism, 6, 10, 49, 68, 86, 100–101, 104, 108

Refugee Act, 85

refugees, 35, 36–8, 85, 116

reification, 17, 26, 56, 109, 121, 123

relationality, 25, 26, 27, 60–61, 68, 119, 124

religion, 13–16, 18, 23, 27, 58

religious fundamentalism, 58

religious iconography, 121

repression, 18, 19, 40–41

reproductive rights, 3, 13; *see also* abortion; contraception

republicanism, 63, 84, 88, 96

responsibility, 24, 31

ressentiment, 56, 58, 129

revolution, 7, 9–11, 19, 48–9, 68, 72, 84–7, 90–91, 95, 100, 108, 117–18, 121

right-wing politics, 58, 102, 107

Rio de Janeiro, 82, 83

ritual, 18, 27, 28

Robinson, Mary, 85

Roche, John, 51

Rose, Kieran, 101–4, 108

RTÉ, 1, 52, 127, 128

Ruane, Lynn, 114

rubber industry, 73–4, 77–9, 83

Ryan, Paul, 38–45, 120

sacramentalism, 18, 27, 30, 67, 87, 88–9

Sapir–Whorf language-thought model, 71

Scott-Heron, Gil, 49

Self, Charles, 51, 62, 65, 96

self harm, 112

Sender, Katherine, 25–6

sex work, 8, 38–46

sexual freedom, 7, 13, 16–20

sexual politics, 29, 46, 54, 72–3, 108

sexual violence, 20, 99

shame, 66–7

Sheehan, Brian, 48

Shonkwiller, Alison, 27

sin, 18, 67

Sinfield, Alan, 82

single mothers, 13

slavery, 73, 74, 79

sleeping sickness, 76, 79

slow violence, 75–6, 79

Smith, Jim, 14–15

social change, 1–2, 6, 49–50, 55, 97, 100–106

social media, 41, 43–4, 67

social partnership, 104–6

social realism, 117

social relations, 16–17, 19, 82, 100, 109, 118, 122

social welfare, 3, 13, 27, 31, 35, 37

socialism, 19, 102, 103

spatiality, 75–6, 83, 118

sport, 42

Steiner, George, 71

stereotyping, 2, 112, 124

stigmatisation, 13, 23, 42, 44, 55, 99, 119

Stonewall, 99

sublimation, 40

subversion, 22, 63

success, 24, 26, 44

suicide, 112–13

Supreme Court, 50–51

surplus repression, 40–41

surplus value, 17, 41

technocracy, 75, 97

temporality, 11, 70, 75–6, 80, 83–4, 110, 121–2, 124–5

terror, 77–9

Thatcher, Margaret, 3

theatre, 61–7

Tiernan, Sonja, 48–50

Time magazine, 1–2, 6, 7

Tóibín, Colm, 85–6

trade unions, 43, 103, 104, 106

Translations (Friel), 71

transphobia, 58

transport, 79–80, 83

Trinity College, 113–14

Two Fuse, 24

unemployment, 3

United Nations, 85

United States, 25, 30–31, 54, 55, 85

universalism, 9, 58, 99, 101, 108

unpaid labour, 17, 28

utopianism, 29, 32, 73, 82, 90, 99, 109–10, 121–2

Varadkar, Leo, 1–7, 29, 94

victimhood, 9, 39, 45, 53, 63, 65

violence, 9, 20, 23, 51–4, 59, 61, 62, 65, 66, 75–80, 90–91, 99

'Viva School of Dance' advertisement, 24, 26, 45, 125

'Volunteers, The' (Caslin), 113–16

vulnerability, 8–9, 28–9, 38, 54–5, 59–68, 88, 90–91, 108, 117–21, 123, 125, 129

wages, 105, 106

Walsh, Eanna, 115

Waterford, 112–13, 119, 121

'We Will Let No Life Be Worth Less' (Fornoff), 114

wealth, 46, 75, 105; *see also* affluence

weddings, 8, 24–9

Weltanschauung, 18

Whelan, Noel, 48

white supremacy, 58

Wilde, Oscar, 72

Williams, Raymond, 21

Williamson, Matthew, 65–7

Women's Right to Choose Campaign, 96, 98

world-systems theory, 105

Yeats, W.B., 70, 89